Schizophrenia - Recent Advances and Patient-Centered Treatment Perspectives

Edited by Jane Yip

Published in London, United Kingdom

Schizophrenia - Recent Advances and Patient-Centered Treatment Perspectives
http://dx.doi.org/10.5772/intechopen.100834
Edited by Jane Yip

Contributors
Bianca Daniela Crecan-Suciu, Ramona Păunescu, Norio Yasui-Furukori, Ryota Yoshida, Kazutaka Shimoda, Akira Imamura, Yoshiro Morimoto, Hitomi Shimizu, Naoki Yamamoto, Hirokazu Kumazaki, Hiroki Ozawa, Tatsiana Dakukina, Victor Obyedkov, Oleg Gorgun, Alexandr Hodjaev, Irina Hvostova, Yulia Kaminskaya, Siarhei Osipchyk, Fedor Khlebokazov, Vera Ivanitskaya, Olga Lapysh, Aliaksandra Kuchynskaya, Ek-Uma Imkome, Inge Nygaard Pedersen, Niels Jørgensen Hannibal, Lars Rye Bertelsen, Lars Ole Bonde, Charlotte Lindvang, Silvia Beatriz Jensen, Nevzat Tarhan, Nesrin Dilbaz, Bahruz Shukurov, Ceylan Ergul, Guner Ulak, Yesim Ozdemir, Türker Tekin Ergüzel, Firdevs Seyfe Sen

First published in London, United Kingdom, 2023 by IntechOpen
IntechOpen is the global imprint of INTECHOPEN LIMITED, registered in England and Wales, registration number: 11086078, 5 Princes Gate Court, London, SW7 2QJ, United Kingdom

British Library Cataloguing-in-Publication Data
A catalogue record for this book is available from the British Library

Additional hard and PDF copies can be obtained from orders@intechopen.com

Schizophrenia - Recent Advances and Patient-Centered Treatment Perspectives
Edited by Jane Yip
p. cm.
Print ISBN 978-1-80355-405-1
Online ISBN 978-1-80355-406-8
eBook (PDF) ISBN 978-1-80355-407-5

Meet the editor

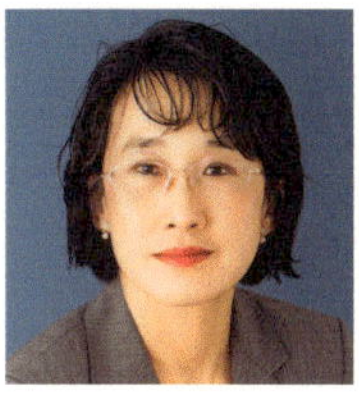

Jane Yip obtained her Ph.D. from the University of Newcastle, Australia, specializing in neuropharmacology. She has worked at Eli Lilly and Company, Indianapolis, USA and has a clinical practice that offers brain mapping and applied behavior analysis (ABA), Indiana Brain Mapping. Her research is on the brain circuit that underlies neurological disorders including depression, autism, and schizophrenia. Although trained in drug development, she has pioneered cutting-edge applications to the treatment of mental disorders from both neurobiology and behavioral science and uses natural environment modification as a treatment approach. She pioneered the use of portable brain imaging to guide behavior treatment for various mental disorders, including schizophrenia. As a member of ABAI and an NGO member of the United Nations, she works on outreach projects in Asia to advance the Universal Declaration of Human Rights, aiming to promote better recognition of individuals with mental disabilities, including schizophrenia. Her overarching aim to is advance treatment intervention, and apply innovative brain-mapping technology to help the public understand mental disorders.

Contents

Preface

When the word "schizophrenia" is mentioned, the public tends to retreat in silent horror. To the lay person, schizophrenia conjures up a spectrum of emotions ranging from fear that a patient will become violent during hallucinatory psychosis, to dismissal that this is a made-up disorder based on a range of normal human emotions that has turned extreme. For some lay audiences, schizophrenia can mean that extreme anxiety has turned into paranoia or that certain traumatic experiences have catapulted a person into a momentary disconnect from reality, and hence they are exhibiting a "psychotic" episode.

In his article in *Psychiatric Times* (November 10, 2021) Dr. Mark Ruffalo, a psychoanalytic psychotherapist at the University of Central Florida College of Medicine and Tufts University School of Medicine, Boston, Massachusetts, explained that schizophrenia is more than an extreme manifestation of what is commonly in the repertoire of human psychology. In his words, there is a misunderstanding that "schizophrenia exists ...... as an extreme variation of normality". It was Paul Blueler (1857–1939) who first introduced the term "schizophrenia" to describe the disorder previously known as Dementia Praecox. According to Dr. Ruffalo, "it is now generally accepted that what we called schizophrenia is likely a grouping of different disease processes, perhaps upward of 200". The dramatic symptoms experienced by patients, their persistence, the degree of impairment, the severity and resistance to being "convinced out of their irrationality" has no parallel in normal mental functioning. Pathological states are a departure from physiological functioning governed by different biological rules or mechanisms of action.

People suffering from the symptoms of schizophrenia often face stigma from society. No research advances can claim success if the knowledge they uncover fails to reach the public and improve their perception of the disorder and its outcomes. Patients suffering from the symptoms of schizophrenia are just like any other person. They deserve to be treated equally, fairly and be fully included in society, which needs to be kind to them and support them in their adversity. By extension, service efforts must incorporate diversity and equity.

Schizophrenia research, like that into any disease, must be committed to integrity and dedicated to partnership with people with the diagnosis, their loved ones, and their community. It goes without saying that research, dissemination, and evidence translation is an international projects that must be dedicated to transparency informed by the highest ethical values.

Educating the next generation of researchers, clinicians, and professionals is essential, as advances in understanding and treatment lie in continual improvement and education. This book collates the latest exciting findings by distinguished researchers, scholars, and professionals who study schizophrenia from various angles; yet their collective works converge into a single mission – exchanging the latest advances in research and facilitating the application of their findings to clinical practice and treatment. The chapters in this book are organized into various topic headings, taking the reader on a journey of understanding schizophrenia through its symptoms and diagnosis, epidemiology, mechanisms of action, brain imaging, psychopharmacology, psycho-behavioral intervention, social inclusion, community care, social action, diversity and inclusion, novel therapeutics and future directions. The rationale for the topics is summarized in brief paragraphs under their respective headings.

This book stands out from similar publications in that it aims to bring a person-and-community-centered approach to a disorder that inflicts a heavy burden not only personally but communally. Patients with schizophrenia and their family as well as members of society must be well informed about the illness so they can form their opinions based on scientific data. Ultimately, the latest research is bringing a message of comfort that improvement in diagnostics, management of clinical trajectories, and therapeutic interventions are not only hope but are coming closer to them as a reality.

To the researchers who have committed their professional lives to the identification, elaboration, discovery, and formulation of the areas of etiology or therapies for schizophrenia, this book brings a multi-disciplinary view so that each researcher can see that, as focused as their own research topic is, it adds to the essential knowledge that demands to be woven into the fabric of understanding of this perplexing human condition called schizophrenia. I hope that the researchers who have contributed to this book will take with them insights from their colleagues from different disciplines and feel, in the spirit of scientific comradeship, that collectively they are moving closer and closer to solving the puzzle of schizophrenia.

Jane Yip
Director,
Indiana Brain Mapping,
Carmel, Indiana, USA

Section 1

Neurobiology

Chapter 1

Neurobiological Perspective and Personalized Treatment in Schizophrenia

Nevzat Tarhan, Nesrin Dilbaz, Bahruz Shukurov, Ceylan Ergul, Guner Ulak, Yesim Ozdemir, Turker Tekin Erguzel and Firdevs Seyfe Sen

Abstract

Personalized treatment is the focus of researchers and comes into prominence for both genetic sciences and neurotechnology. Recently, clinical practice tries to follow the idea and principles of personalized medicine. Besides predicting an individual's sensibility or predisposition for developing schizophrenia, pharmacogenetic and pharmacogenomic approaches attempt to define and acknowledge important indicators of clinical response to antipsychotics namely their efficacy and adverse effects. Particularly in the treatment of schizophrenia, clinicians are very helpless in resistant cases, and clinical pharmacogenomics contributes in a revolutionary way. With both phenotyping, namely Therapeutic Drug Monitoring (TDM) and genotyping, "big expectations" emerged both with the right drug, the right dose, and the right time. Both pharmacokinetic genotyping, CYP400 enzyme activity, and pharmacodynamic genotyping could be measured. The chapter handles schizophrenia with neurobiological views and covers personalized treatment approaches from various perspectives. Personalized treatment in the diagnosis and treatment of schizophrenia is presented first. Following comorbid schizophrenia in addition to the use of various substances, psychopharmacology of schizophrenia and the mechanism of action of antipsychotic drugs are presented. Genetics and epigenetics in schizophrenia are studied in detail and *in silico* application and computational approaches covering the feature extraction process and destructive impact of the metaverse are shared lastly.

Keywords: neuromodulation, tTMS, dTMS, pharmacogenetic, psycopharmacology, addiction, drug interactions, therapeutic drug monitoring, personalized medicine, personalized treatment, neuroimaging, deep learning, metaverse, entropy, genetics and epigenetics

1. Introduction

Rapidly evolving MRI technologies and their multimodal combinations provide biological findings that allow support for various hypotheses attempting to explain

IntechOpen

schizophrenia. PET and SPECT techniques have been used to study neurotransmitter mechanisms. Magnetic resonance spectroscopy has demonstrated neurochemical changes in vivo in patients with schizophrenia, As a result, we better understand the detailed brain anatomy, pathophysiology, and chemical pathology of schizophrenia. More importantly, findings from neuroimaging studies promise to transform existing diagnostic tools into new functional tools with implications for the treatment of patients. Accumulating data from genome-wide association studies are constantly decoding SZ risk genes. Especially with the widespread use of new generation sequencing systems, it has been shown that more than 200 loci may play a role in the etiology. In addition, epigenetic factors should not be forgotten. Biomarker studies(BDNF,MB-COMT, COMT, RELN and HTR2 etc.) have proven that DNA methylation and histone acetylation are also effective in the development of schizophrenia. The use of epigenetic treatments in practice and the development of gene therapy options provide hope for the treatment of such neuropsychiatric diseases. Targets of psychopharmacology include positive symptoms, negative symptoms, mood symptoms, cognitive deficits, life quality and occupational functionalities. Choice is usually guided by the target symptom and depends on the pharmacotherapy of the drug. Typical and atypical antipsychotic medications are gold standard in the management of the disease. Unfortunately, at the present day there is no obvious or best choice of drug in antipsychotic medication. Several G protein-coupled receptors (GPCRs), mainly dopamine, serotonin and adrenaline receptors are traditional molecular targets for psychopharmacological strategies of schizophrenia. Thus, drug development efforts now target novel important signaling mechanisms of GPCRs. Since the treatment of schizophrenia addresses the phenotype and not the cause, and our current knowledge about the illness is not enough, the pharmacotherapy of schizophrenia is far to yield promising results. There has been a large literature and experience with theoretical neuromodulations such as rTMS, dTMS. With the involvement and applications of artificial intelligence in medical data, patient follow-up strategies and methodologies are likely to happen in the near future. This study focusses on the strategies in this perspective and underline the personalized treatment for the diagnosis and treatment of schizophrenia. Since schizophrenia is in the scope of various disciplines like medicine, pharmacology, biology and natural sciences the chapter is structured and studied with the support of the aforementioned titles of those disciplines.

2. Personalized treatment in the diagnosis and treatment of schizophrenia

In recent years, personalized treatments have come to the fore, both in genetic sciences and developments in neurotechnological discoveries. Especially in the treatment of schizophrenia (SZ), clinicians are very helpless in resistant cases. No new pharmacological agents have been found in the last decade. However, clinical pharmacogenomic developments have revolutionarily come to the rescue. With both phenotyping, Therapeutic Drug Monitoring (TDM) and genotyping, great advantages have emerged in terms of the right drug, the right dose and the right time. Both pharmacokinetic genotyping, CYP400 enzyme activity and pharmacodynamic genotyping, namely Catechol-O-methyltransferase (COMT) and the serotonin transporter (5-HTT) enzyme activity, can be easily measured. On the other hand, a great deal of literature knowledge and experience has been shared regarding noninvasive neuromodulation treatments with high reliability in treatment, such as repetitive transcranial magnetic stimulation (rTMS) and deep transcranial magnetic stimulation (dTMS). Moreover, it is possible to create patient follow-up systems by combining artificial intelligence and medical records. It is necessary to consider all this information in more detail.

2.1 Phenotyping

TDM is a new method for optimizing drug therapy. The aim is to understand the plasma concentrations of psychoactive drugs and discuss how efficiently they can be applied in psychiatry practice in patient safety and treatment-resistant situations. TDM is based on the principle that there is a close relationship between the plasma level of the drug and its clinical effect. If such a relationship does not exist TDM is of little value. TDM as a preliminary test for genetic polymorphisms;

- Improves therapeutic efficacy,
- Improves drug safety,
- Reduces total therapeutic costs,
- To get results in two days, cheap cost

Psychoactive drugs are divided into four groups for drug blood level monitoring. First, strongly recommended drugs for toxicity monitoring such as lithium, carbamazepine, valproic acid. Second, Follow-up for side-effect control; like clozapine. Third, the ones followed for the anticipation of drug response include drugs that do not want to waste time with trial and testing. And lastly, it is used for the preliminary diagnosis of genetic polymorphism in treatment-resistant cases and for the decision of appropriate drug selection. Genetic Polymorphism can be determined by Genetic Profiling (DNA tests) and is a very valuable parameter for Personalized Medicine. It is very important for the patient's treatment compliance that we can predict the reduced drug effect, increased drug side-effects and toxicity risk. Why is it important to identify genes and proteins related to Gene Polymorphism that might have very important clinical results? Tests for drug efficacy and patient safety are important for the principle of the appropriate drug, dose, and duration. Clinical Pharmacogenetics, which deals with DNA sequence analysis and drug blood level monitoring together, has started an important period in Psychiatry. Knowing the genetic and pharmacological basis of the diversity seen in human response to drugs is no longer a mere scientific curiosity. Follow-up of side effects at the recommended dose, lack of clinical response, and drug interactions have different importance in children and the elderly (see in **Figure 1**) [1].

2.2 Genotyping

In order to predict the possibility of the patient experiencing toxicity, when monitoring medication level increases and decreases are imperative. In order to produce important clinical results, it is important to understand gene polymorphisms. Combining the analysis of psychiatric DNA series and therapeutic drug

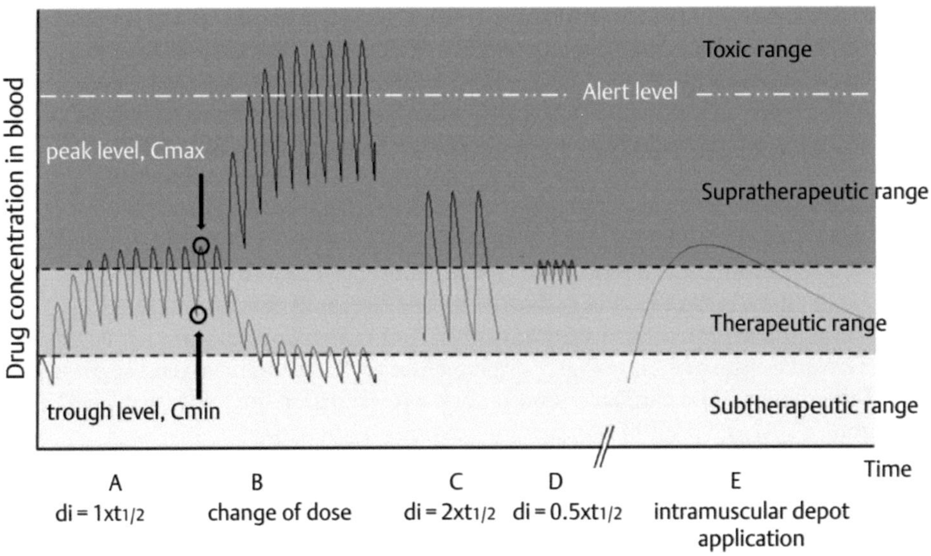

Figure 1.
It is recommended to increase atypical or typical antipsychotics such as clozapine, olanzapine, risperidone, and paliperidone to supratherapeutic level in treatment-resistant SZ cases. Concentration time curve after oral or intramuscular depot medication. A: 94% of steady state (therapy with constant dose) is reached after four elimination half-lives (t1/2) of the drug. At steady-state, drug intake equals drug elimination over a defined time frame. Trough levels at steady state are usually quantified and recommended for TDM. The figure shows a hypothetical drug with a dosing interval (di) equal to its half-life (di = t1/2), a situation found similar for many drugs (e.g., t1/2 = 12 h, di = 12 h, curve A). Trough concentrations are right in the middle of the therapeutic range, i.e., on target, despite the fact that the drug's concentrations during the dosing interval sometimes exceed the therapeutic range. B: Modification of drug concentrations by doubling or halving the dose without change of the dosing interval. C: Doubling the dose interval (di = 2 × t1/2) and administering the entire daily dose once daily results in curve C. The area under the blood concentration versus time curve (AUC) representing the total drug exposition is identical for curves A and C, however, trough concentrations in curve C (24 h after the daily dose) are significantly lower than in curve A (12 h after a half daily dose). High differences between trough and peak levels can be associated with tolerability problems during the phases of high drug concentrations. D: Curve D illustrates the intake of four equal doses per day, resulting in the same daily dose as for curves A to C. Again, the AUC is identical to curves A and C but this time we observe higher trough concentrations. Using this application form, even low doses can be effective, since sufficient drug concentrations are available at the target structures. E: Intramuscular application of depot: Peak concentrations may be achieved after as early as 1 day or as late as 4 weeks depending on the formulation. Concentrations comparable to trough values after oral application can only be obtained immediately prior to the next application. Blood sampling during the elimination phase after full absorption (maximum) will result in higher values compared to trough sampling after oral application despite equal AUC. Please note the time scale for curve E is different from curves A to D [1].

monitoring, clinical pharmacogenomics has started a new era in which patients are provided with a personalized pharmaceutical treatment. So, genotyping findings give us the power of predictability in drug selection based on gene variations (see in **Table 1**).

In **Table 2**, a pharmacogenomic profile is seen regarding which drug to be administered in a genotyping case. Genotyping; works for specific mutations, provides information about metabolic capacity, only one-time oral sampling is enough, results stay valid a life time (Pharmacogenetic ID). Measuring COMT enzyme activity is another genotyping method in order to estimate the effect of antipsychotic drugs on the Pharmacodynamics, namely the Central Nervous System. If COMT enzyme activity is slow, less and delayed response should be expected. Neuromodulation treatment indication and supratherapeutic drug dose should be considered. Measuring COMT

	CYP1A2	CYP2C9	CYP2C19	CYP2D6	CYP3A4
Substrate	Clozapine	N/A	N/A	Risperidone Haloperidol	Quetiapine
Inhibitor	N/A	N/A	N/A	Haloperidol	N/A

Abbreviations: N/A: Not Applicable, Cytochrome P450 1A2 (CYP1A2).

Table 1.
Example of predictability in drug selection based on gene variations by Tarhan.

Gene	Phenotyping	Enzime activity
CYP1A2	UM	Increased
CYP2C9	UMdim	Decreased
CYP2C19	EM	Normal
CYP2D6	PM	Decreased

Abbreviations: EM: Extensive metabolizer, EM dim: Extensive metabolizer, diminished, PM: Poor Metabolizer, UM: Ultra-rapid metabolizer, Cytochrome P450 1A2 (CYP1A2), Cytochrome P450 family 2 subfamily C member 9 (CYP2C9), Cytochrome P450 subfamily C member 19 (CYP2C19), Cytochrome P450 family 2 subfamily D member 6 (CYP2D6).

Table 2.
Example of genes, phenotyping and enzyme activity by Tarhan.

enzyme activity is another genotyping method in order to estimate the effect of antipsychotic drugs on the Pharmacodynamics, namely the Central Nervous System. If COMT enzyme activity is slow, less and delayed response should be expected. Neuromodulation treatment indication and supratherapeutic drug dose should be considered. COMT is responsible for the O-methylation of catecholamines, chemical compounds derived from the amino acid tyrosine [2]. Although the structural organization of COMT is currently conceptualized as a single gene, this single gene encodes two similar enzymes. One is soluble and is called S-COMT. The other is membrane bound and called MB-COMT. A well-known genetic variation of COMT was described more than 30 years ago [3]. This genetic variation was called as the Val 158Met polymorphism for many years, referring to an amino acid change at position 158th in the amino acid sequence of the membrane-bound form of the enzyme. It is also less commonly referred to as 472G/A. This functional polymorphism has been assigned a unique reference sequence number, rs4680 now. Val allele of rs4680 (guanine allele) is a more active allele than Met allele (adenine allele) and has been accepted as a risk factor for SZ [4–7]. In summary, the introduction of genetic profile monitoring into routine psychiatric practice in TDM and resistant cases, which is a faster and easier method, seems to be a revolutionary development. Certainly, the availability of special tests for personalized treatment has been the greatest contribution of science to the clinic.

3. Comorbid schizophrenia in addiction

Alcohol and substance use disorders (ASUD) is a diagnostic group that has been shown to frequently accompany other mental illnesses in many epidemiological studies [5]. One of these mental illnesses is psychotic disorders, and a well-known example is SZ. Addiction and SZ are both chronic disorders with serious consequences both at the individual and the public level. Substance use in SZ as "self-medication" is presented as a hypothesis, suggesting that substances are used to control or alleviate the symptoms of SZ. This hypothesis claims to predict the selection of the substance used according to the present symptom. For example, patients with SZ may be expected to use stimulants for their negative symptoms. In reality, stimulant abuse is not common in SZ, and many studies do not support this hypothesis. People with SZ often tend to abuse easily accessible substances. Reasons for use are similar to those of the general population ('to get high', 'to reduce depression', 'to relax'). The symptoms that are most commonly associated with addiction in patients with SZ are depressive symptoms [6]. The brain reward center theory proposed by Green et al. has received much support for explaining the high frequency of substance use disorders seen in patients with SZ. This theory proposes that there is an abnormality in dopamine-mediated responses in the brain to reward stimuli in individuals with a diagnosis of SZ [7]. Based on animal and human studies, this abnormality is thought to occur secondary to front striatal and limbic structure abnormality in the brain reward center [8]. The lifetime prevalence of addiction in the general population is 16%. On the other hand, even when nicotine use is excluded, nearly half of SZ patients are diagnosed with a lifelong substance use disorder. The Epidemiological Field Study reports that 34% of patients with SZ have alcohol use disorder and 28% have a substance use disorder [5]. Data from the National Epidemiological Study of Alcohol and Related Conditions revealed that SZ is associated with an increased risk for reuse, especially when cannabis is involved [9]. When we take nicotine into consideration, comorbidity rates will increase significantly. Exacerbation of psychotic symptoms, relapse and hospitalization, use of emergency services, HIV, HCV, HBV infections, suicidal behavior and homelessness have been associated with an increased risk of substance abuse in patients with a diagnosis of SZ. These patients with dual diagnoses also have a worse prognosis for other concomitant medical problems such as diabetes mellitus. Addiction comorbidity in patients with SZ seems to be associated with violence and criminal behavior. Substance use in patients with SZ is most often not questioned, screened, or diagnosed. Roughly half of SZ patients can be considered to have an addiction-related problem. Asking about current and also lifelong substance use is a part of psychiatric examination, and this subject should be discussed with every SZ patient [10–12]. Substances used among SZ patients are as follows (in order of frequency): nicotine, alcohol, cannabis and cocaine. The frequency of alcohol use disorder is three, and the substance use disorders is five times higher in patients with SZ compared with the general population. Abuse of more than one substance is quite common in this population. Although nicotine use tends to decrease in the general population, it has been observed at constant rates in the SZ population for over 40 years. Patients with SZ use amphetamines, opioids, and sedative-hypnotics less frequently [12].

3.1 Schizophrenia and smoking

21% of the normal population and 72–90% of patients diagnosed with SZ smoke. Smokers with SZ are addicted to more nicotine than the general population, are more commonly diagnosed with medical illnesses, and less frequently seek help to quit smoking. Negative symptoms such as apathy, positive symptoms such as disorganized thinking, and cognitive impairment reduce both the motivation to quit smoking and the compliance to implement smoking cessation strategies. On the other hand, smoking also negatively affects antipsychotic drug treatments. Smoking increases the efficiency of the Cytochrome P450 1A2 (CYP1A2) microsomal enzyme system, which is involved in the metabolism of some antipsychotics, especially haloperidol, phenothiazines, clozapine and olanzapine. This may explain the need to use antipsychotics at higher doses in smokers with SZ compared to nonsmokers [13–15].

3.2 Schizophrenia and alcohol use

Studies show that 25–45% of patients with SZ use alcohol at a level that fulfills the criteria of alcohol use disorder [16, 17]. It has been reported that patients with SZ who have comorbid alcohol use disorder have more severe symptoms, are hospitalized more frequently, and have worse long-term treatment outcomes [18].

3.3 Schizophrenia and cannabis use

Cannabis use rates in people with SZ vary between %27 and %42, and these rates are higher than those of the general population [18]. In a follow-up study on cannabis use and the development of SZ, a six-fold higher risk of developing SZ was found in those who reported more than fifty times of cannabis use in lifetime [19]. It has been reported that the etiological relationship between cannabis use and SZ spectrum disorder is related to cannabinoid receptors and some genetic polymorphisms. The cannabinoid 1 (CB-1) receptor is associated with a group of neurotransmitter systems that play a role in the etiology of SZ, such as the dopaminergic and glutamatergic systems. Specific differences have been shown in the regional density of CB-1 receptors in the brains of patients who developed psychosis after cannabis use [20]. In another study conducted on adolescents using cannabis, it was determined that having a functional polymorphism in the COMT gene was a moderate risk factor for the onset of psychosis. It has been reported that the risk of developing psychosis with cannabis use is high in individuals carrying the COMT gene Val-158 allele [21].

3.4 Schizophrenia and cocaine use

Studies have reported that between 15% and 50% of SZ patients use cocaine [16, 22]. It has been reported that cocaine can reduce the negative symptoms of SZ and is often used to relieve depression [23]. It is also known that cocaine causes an increase in dopamine concentration at the synaptic junction, thus increasing Dopamine 1 and Dopamine 2 (D1 and D2) receptor activities, and thus may cause psychotic symptoms in users [24].

3.5 Schizophrenia and stimulant use

While clinical experience indicates that amphetamine psychosis can last for a maximum of 3–6 months, there is insufficient evidence that this substance will directly cause SZ. However, if the individual has SZ sensitivity, it can be proposed that amphetamines used in high doses increase the risk of SZ. Results of a Finnish national study found an 8-year cumulative risk of 30% for a diagnosis of a spectrum of SZ in individuals presenting with amphetamine-induced psychosis [25]. It is reported that approximately 26–46% of individuals with methamphetamine addiction have amphetamine-induced psychosis [26]. Symptoms of methamphetamine-related psychosis are similar to those of paranoid SZ. Auditory hallucinations, persecutory and reference delusions are common. Negative symptoms appear relatively rarely, and the process is quite heterogeneous [12].

3.6 Schizophrenia and hallucinogen use

There is not sufficient evidence that Lysergic acid diethylamide (LSD) causes prolonged psychotic symptoms. The frequency of hallucinogen-induced psychosis changing to a diagnosis in the SZ spectrum during eight years has been reported as %24. The most common diagnosis is schizoaffective disorder, and mood symptoms are present [12].

3.7 Schizophrenia and opioid use

The Epidemiological Field Study found more associations between opioid use disorders and SZ than previous studies [5]. The CATIE study, on the other hand, found low levels of opioid abuse or dependence in participants with SZ [27]. In the 1970s, an investigation of methadone causing elevated prolactin levels demonstrated its dopamine-blocking effect. The inhibition of adenylate cyclase by antipsychotic drugs such as haloperidol, similar to methadone and other opioids, has led to the theory that opioid agonists have antipsychotic effects. The combined use of methadone and neuroleptics in the treatment of SZ was investigated in the 1980s. In a study conducted with a limited number of SZ patients, it was reported that methadone added to chlorpromazine had a moderate but statistically significant effect on psychotic symptoms [28]. In a study conducted in 1998, it was reported that individuals with a history of mental illness who stated that they did not use opioids in the baseline used more opioids after a 3-year follow-up than those who did not have a history of mental illness [29]. Although it is known that people with a psychiatric history use opioids more frequently, limited data is of the relation with psychotic disorders.

3.8 Schizophrenia and use of other substances

Abuse of anticholinergic drugs has been reported primarily in patients with a psychiatric diagnosis [30]. It is unclear whether patients use these drugs to treat their extrapyramidal symptoms or to treat their negative symptoms. It has been reported that the negative symptoms of schizophrenic patients with anticholinergic drug abuse are more dominant, and this supports the theory that cholinergic hyperactivity has a significant effect on the negative symptoms of SZ [31]. There is limited information about the use of other substances in patients with SZ. In a study by Warner et al., the rate of inhalant use in individuals with SZ was found to be 29.1% [32].

3.9 Treatment

Carrying out the appropriate treatment for both diseases by the same treatment team will also allow the continuation of outpatient treatment in the long term. According to neurobiological approaches, dysfunction in the brain reward circuit should be targeted to reduce substance use in patients with SZ. In addition to drug therapy, general and specific psychotherapeutic, socio-therapeutic and occupational therapy should also be applied. General principles of treatment for intoxication and withdrawal can also be applied to patients who are diagnosed with SZ.

However, if the patient continues to receive antipsychotic treatment, drug interactions should be taken into consideration. Benzodiazepines should be preferred, especially in alcohol withdrawal syndrome, because they show fewer interactions and prevent seizures that may develop due to withdrawal and delirium [33–35]. It is not necessary to use higher doses of antipsychotics in the treatment of psychotic symptoms compared to patients without substance use disorder comorbidity. Although high doses of antipsychotics successfully treat psychotic symptoms, they seem far from eliminating the psychokinetic effects of the substances. Recent reviews in schizophrenic patients with substance abuse indicate that second-generation antipsychotics (SGAs) are superior to first-generation antipsychotics (FGAs) because of their different receptor profiles. There is limited data showing that FGAs reduce substance abuse in patients with SZ, whereas there is data showing that haloperidol treatment increases the rate of smoking in patients with SZ [36]. Clozapine seems to be the most appropriate treatment for SZ patients with comorbid substance use disorders. It has been shown that clozapine decreases the craving for cocaine use [37], the rate of smoking [38], the rate of substance use [38–42], and increases the number of days without drugs [40, 41]. The level of evidence regarding the effectiveness of other atypical antipsychotics on substance use is still weak. Cases of quetiapine abuse have been reported, and it should be questioned if it is being used according to the prescription [42]. In the treatment of alcohol use disorder accompanying SZ, a limited number of studies in which naltrexone, disulfiram, and Acamprosate were added to antipsychotic treatment showed that these treatments were well tolerated and had a positive effect [33]. Using psychopharmacological agents in the smoking cessation treatment of patients with SZ may be more frequently required compared to the general population. Nicotine replacement therapies can be used alone or in combination with a therapy method, bupropion and varenicline, and can be used effectively and reliably in patients with dual diagnoses [43]. Substances used can affect the effectiveness of antipsychotic treatments. Smoking causes a decrease in blood levels of haloperidol, fluphenazine, olanzapine and clozapine [44]. Quitting smoking will cause an increase in drug blood levels. On the other hand, caffeine acts as a competitive inhibitor for CYP1A2, which acts in the metabolism of antipsychotics. Therefore, caffeine increases the blood levels of antipsychotics such as olanzapine and clozapine [45]. All substance use disorders, especially cocaine, accompanying SZ increase the possibility of extrapyramidal side effects due to antipsychotic drugs [46].

4. Psychopharmacology of schizophrenia

SZ is a chronic, often debilitating, and relapsing mental disorder, approximately with a lifetime prevalence near 1% [47]. Relatively specific core symptoms of SZ manifest as a combination of positive symptoms (hallucinations, delusions, impaired thinking, disorganized behavior) negative symptoms (affective blunting, emotional withdrawal, poverty of speech, anhedonia and apathy) and/or cognitive impairment (learning, memory, attention and executive functions deficits) [48]. Typical and atypical antipsychotic medications are gold standard in the management of the disease. An essential difference between typical and atypical antipsychotics is that, atypical antipsychotics with lower affinity [49] and faster dissociation rate [50] at the dopamine D2 receptor, may cause minimal extrapyramidal side effects (EPS) or prolactin elevation, decreased cognitive impairment and greater improvement in negative symptoms although there are some exceptions [50]. Since treatment of negative symptoms and cognitive disorders keep on being a serious problem by current antipsychotic drugs, and positive symptoms are resistant to currently available medications in a substantial number of patients, it challenges the researches to investigate more effective and better-tolerated novel targets used as either monotherapies or as adjunctive treatments added to currently available antipsychotics [51]. The use of adjunctive pharmacological agents might offer a viable approach for cognitive functions since they can be used to modulate specific neurotransmitter systems hypothesized to be associated with cognitive functions. Unfortunately, at the present day there is no obvious or best choice of drug in antipsychotic medication.

4.1 Mechanism of action of antipsychotic drugs

SZ involves alterations of dopamine neurotransmission in brain circuits with excess dopaminergic activity in the mesolimbic pathway responsible for positive symptoms and reduced dopaminergic signaling in the mesocortical pathway causing negative symptoms, complemented by the glutamatergic hypothesis which considers changes in prefrontal neuronal connectivity involving glutamatergic neurotransmission at NMDA receptor [52]. Thus, the antagonism of D2 receptors in the mesolimbic pathway will produce reductions in dopamine activity and psychotic symptoms [53]. All known antipsychotic drugs (APDs) with documented efficacy on positive psychotic symptoms have affinity for the D2 receptor and fully or partially block the actions of dopamine [54]. D2 receptors mediate their physiological actions through both G-protein dependent and independent signaling [55]. Thus, drug development efforts now target novel important signaling mechanisms of G protein-coupled receptors (GPCRs) mainly dopaminergic, serotonergic, cholinergic, glutamatergic, adenosine and other neurotransmitter systems.

4.2 Dopaminergic mechanisms

All APDs increase the turnover and the release of dopamine as a consequence of postsynaptic dopamine receptor blockade in certain brain regions. The three principal dopaminergic pathways in the brain play role in the antipsychotic activity of antipsychotic drugs to different extends: The nigrostriatal pathway is considered to be responsible for extrapyramidal symptoms and cognitive function, in addition long-term blockade of this pathway may cause up-regulation resulting with tardive dyskinesia; The mesolimbic pathway is thought to be involved in delusion and hallucinations of psychosis, emotional activity, reward and motivation (blockade of D2 receptors in this pathway is thought to mediate the antipsychotic efficacy of the antipsychotic drug and its ability to reduce or block positive symptoms); The mesocortical pathway is thought to be involved in the production of positive and negative psychotic symptoms and cognitive processing (blockade of D2 receptors in this pathway may produce blunting of emotions and cognitive side effects, limiting the negative symptoms of SZ [56, 57]. It should be pointed out that antipsychotic effect necessitates the modulation of D2 receptors. All APDs are mixed D2/D3 and often also Dopamine 4 (D4) ligands with Dopamine (D3) and D4 subtypes having attractive limbic/cortical expression pattern. No evidence exists supporting the efficacy of a selective D3 antagonist by itself on psychotic symptoms, but it may enhance the efficacy of D2 antagonism and reduce EPS potential [48].

4.3 Serotonergic mechanisms

Serotonin 2A (5-HT2A) antagonism is the most investigated mechanism since it is the main driver of atypicality [58]. Atypical antipsychotics almost always have higher affinity for 5HT2A receptors than they do for D2 receptors. 5-HT2A receptor blockade along with weaker D2 receptor blockade may play role in the ability of atypical APDs to increase dopamine levels in the medial prefrontal cortex while exerting weaker effect on limbic dopamine efflux. This may contribute to their advantages for cognition, negative symptoms and antipsychotic activity. Partial agonist actions at 5HT1A receptors and partial agonist actions at D2 receptors in addition to 5HT2A antagonism, can also mediate the atypical antipsychotic clinical profile of low EPS and less hyperprolactinemia with comparable antipsychotic actions [51, 56, 57]. Blocking 5HT2C receptors stimulates dopamine and norepinephrine release in prefrontal cortex, and has pro-cognitive but particularly antidepressant actions. Some atypical APDs have potent 5-HT2C-antagonist activity, including those with known antidepressant action (e.g. quetiapine and olanzapine [59].

A few APDs have moderate affinity for (and partial agonist activity at) 5-HT1A receptors (e.g., clozapine, ziprasidone, quetiapine and aripiprazole). Atypical APDs with either potent 5HT2A antagonism or potent 5HT1A agonist/partial agonist properties, or with both actions, have a reduced incidence of EPS and thought to improve negative symptoms and cognitive impairment [51, 57, 59]. Serotonin 2C (5-HT2C) antagonism may contribute to weight gain induced by several atypical APDs [2] while Serotonin IA (5-HT1A) agonism may be responsible for reducing the potential for weight gain of atypical APDs [57].

4.4 Adrenergic receptors

All atypical antipsychotic has at least moderate binding potency to α1-adrenergic receptors which contributes to their side effects. α1 antagonist activity may have implications for lowering EPS. Several atypical antipsychotics also have α2 antagonist properties and attenuation of inhibition of noradrenergic and serotonergic neurons by α2 antagonists is believed to improve mood and may contribute to the beneficial effects of antipsychotics on mood [51, 56, 59].

4.5 Acetylcholine receptors

Blockade of muscarinic receptors by some APDs are useful in the treatment of SZ especially by limiting EPS. However, affinity for the muscarinic receptor results with increase in unacceptable autonomic side effects and differences in affinity for the muscarinic receptor subtypes significantly affects the properties of the drug. Muscarinic antagonists used for treating EPS have been reported to ameliorate negative symptoms of SZ [13] while muscarinic M1 receptor agonism might be beneficial in treating the cognitive dysfunction as well as the psychotic symptoms in SZ [60].

4.6 Drug development strategies

Since several different elements of the neural circuitry underlie the multiple deficits of SZ, treatment requires drugs acting through different mechanisms. Comprehensive research on GPCRs resulted in the exploration of novel important signaling mechanisms of GPCRs which are crucial for drug discovery. It seems rational to develop molecules having a little affinity to D2 receptors and also binding to one or more preferred targets such as 5-HT1A, 5-HT2A, 5-HT2C, 5-HT6, 5-HT7, glutamatergic and/or nicotinergic receptors, while avoiding interaction of targets such as α1-adrenergic, H1, M1 and M3 receptor activity. To design single-target agents that can be used to augment multi-target agents is another option in APD development. Single-target vs. multi-target agents will likely remain at the main point of APD development. Since cognitive deficits in SZ are widely prevalent and appear to be correlated with social and occupational function, improving cognitive function should be a characteristic of all newly developed drugs used for the treatment of SZ [54, 61].

4.7 Dopaminergic targets

Since D2 receptor has been the 'Holy Grail' for the development of APDs, pharmacologic initiatives to reduce neurotransmission through the D2 receptor represent the only proven therapeutic mechanism for psychoses. D1 receptor antagonist or agonist, D2 receptor partial agonist, D3 receptor antagonist and D4 receptor antagonist molecules are new targets of drug development for APDs. The newest novel group of antipsychotic drugs, aripiprazole, brexpiprazole and cariprazine unlike others, are not dopamine. D2 receptor antagonists but D2 partial agonists [62]. The D3 receptors, with similar properties as D2 receptors, appear to be promising candidates for antipsychotic drug discovery. D5 receptors, with similar properties with D1 receptors have attracted attention for the treatment of cognitive disturbances, with an effect likely mediated through enhancement of NMDA receptor function [48, 57].

4.8 Serotonergic targets

5-HT3 receptors regulate inhibitory Gamma Aminobutyric Acid (GABA) interneurons in various brain areas that in turn regulate the release of a number of neurotransmitters. Blocking 5-HT3 receptors on GABA interneurons increases the release of serotonin, dopamine, norepinephrine, acetylcholine and histamine in the cortex and is thus a novel approach to a pro-cognitive agent [57]. 5-HT4 receptors, expressed in nigrostriatal and mesolimbic systems, can modulate the release of Ach, dopamine, GABA and serotonin. 5-HT4 receptors may be an attractive target for improving cognition in SZ, since currently available atypical ASDs generally lack significant affinity for 5-HT4 receptors [63]. 5-HT6 receptor antagonists have been proposed as novel adjunct targets for antipsychotics in enhancing cognitive function and/or treating negative symptoms in SZ [57, 64]. 5HT7 receptors, important regulators of serotonin release, exert significant roles in circadian rhythms, mood and sleep. Several APDs are 5HT7 antagonists and may have important roles in learning and memory [57].

4.9 Glutamatergic targets

Glutamatergic system, particularly by antagonizing NMDA sensitive glutamate receptors, is another neurotransmitter system underlying pathogenesis of SZ. Under activity of the mesocortical dopamine system may mediate the negative, cognitive and affective symptoms of SZ and could also be linked to hypo functioning of NMDA receptors at different GABA interneurons. Thus, disturbances in glutamate signaling may be an attractive drug target for SZ due to its key role in the path mechanism of this disease especially in regards of cognitive impairment and negative symptoms [65, 66]. The glycine regulatory site agonists (e.g. glycine-cyclomerized-serine and D-alanine) are potential targets for APD development since they augment NMDA-receptor mediated activity. Metabotropic glutamate receptor (mGluR),another class of glutamate receptor, presynaptic antagonists/postsynaptic agonists may provide a new alternative monotherapy for the treatment of SZ [57, 67]. α-amino-3-hydroxy-5-methyl-4-isoxazolepropionic acid (AMPA) receptors are glutamate receptor subtypes, leading to NMDA receptor activation. Ampakines, a class of compounds that enhance receptor function, represent another potential target for treatment of SZ with expectance of more efficacy for cognitive symptoms and without exerting activation of positive symptoms or neurotoxicity [57, 68]. Since glycine transporter inhibitors (GlyT1 e.g. sarcosine, bitopertin) increase NMDA neurotransmission, it is expected that they will be able to adequately reduce the hypo functioning of NMDA receptors in order to lead improvement, especially in the negative and cognitive symptoms of SZ, perhaps also augment the improvement in positive symptoms achieved by treatment with atypical antipsychotics, and thus attract maximum overall efficacy in SZ [56, 69]. Glutathione precursor (N-acetylcysteine) could be also be of clinical benefit in the treatment of SZ by preventing oxidative stress and enhancing neurotransmission at NMDA-receptors [53, 70].

4.10 Other aminergic GPCR targets

Besides dopamine and serotonin receptors, other aminergic receptors i.e., adrenergic, cholinergic, muscarinic and histaminergic receptors are also linked to SZ. Potential benefits of α2-adrenergic receptor agonists or antagonists in SZ remains unclear. α7 nicotinic, acetylcholine (ach) receptor agonists (3-2,4-dimethoxybenzylidene anabaseine, tropisetron) and α4-β2 nicotinic receptor agonists (varenicline) are possible adjunctive targets to APDs for the treatment SZ [54]. Modulation of dopamine and glutamatergic neurons by cholinergic muscarinic receptors (e.g. muscarinic M1/M4 agonist xanomeline) has been new targets of APD development [60, 71]. Results of attempts aiming to increase ach receptors concentration and potential activity at both nicotinic and muscarinic receptors by Ach esterase inhibitors for improving cognitive function in SZ are controversial [51]. There is a correlation between increased histamine occupancy and decreased cognitive performance. Antipsychotics have moderate antagonistic potency for H1 receptors with some exceptions [59]. H3receptor antagonists/inverse agonists are targets of drug researches as a possibly novel class of drugs with precognitive properties [53, 72]. Molecules avoiding H1 receptor affinity and 5-HT2C antagonism might be useful in preventing antipsychotic-induced sedation and weight gain [73].

4.11 Other targets

Agents that increase GABAergic inhibition of cortical pyramidal cells have been hypothesized to improve working memory and other cognitive impairments in SZ. Phosphodiesterase (PDE) inhibitors, improve neurotransmission by affecting intracellular second messenger signaling and particularly PDE2, PDE4, PDE5 and PDE10 inhibitors seem promising for treating cognitive symptoms of SZ [27]. Neurokinin-3 (NK3) tachykinin receptor antagonist (osanetant, talnetant), estrogen, oxytocin, secretin, erythropoietin, neuroactive steroids, omega-3 fatty acids and ginkgo are adjunctive candidate modulators of SZ. Complementary minocycline, anti-inflammatory agents (celecoxib) and COMT inhibitors (tolcapone, entacapone) might have benefit effects in SZ and it is postulated that immunotherapy is a treatment option for this syndrome [74]. Already there exists numerous updated guidelines for the pharmacological treatment of patients with SZ although consistent and contradictory recommendations exist between them [75]. The discovery of effective novel therapeutic agents for the treatment of SZ will require our understanding of the molecular and functional pathophysiological mechanisms playing role in SZ.

Since several different elements of the neural circuitry underlie the multiple deficits of SZ, radical new approaches require a deeper understanding of the path mechanism and causes of the disorder that are still insufficiently understood. Although D2 antagonist/partial agonist properties can explain the antipsychotic efficacy for positive symptoms as well as many side effects of antipsychotics, and the 5HT2A antagonist, 5HT1A partial agonist and muscarinic antagonist properties can explain the reduced propensity for EPS or elevating prolactin by various antipsychotics, many additional pharmacologic properties of these drugs also play role. Glutamatergic system, particularly by antagonizing NMDA sensitive glutamate receptors, is an attractive neurotransmitter system affecting psychosis in SZ. Cholinergic, muscarinic, GABA and glutamate receptors also play role in the psychotherapy of SZ. They are capable to modulate antipsychotic drug action, including EPS and cognition, through several direct and indirect mechanisms. Current efforts in drug design against SZ focus on cognitive behavioral psychotherapy in order to strengthen the patient's capacity for normal thinking using mental exercises and self-observation besides searching for compounds treating negative symptoms and as well as better tolerated. We are aimed to overview of different strategies and targets under investigation for the development of novel psychological therapies in the treatment of SZ involving mainly novel mechanisms of GPCRs signaling.

5. Genetics and epigenetics in schizophrenia

SZ is a severe mental-psychiatric disorder for which there is no definite knowledge about its underlying mechanisms. Although the complex interactions of genetic and environmental factors play a role in the etiology of SZ, studies on twins have shown that hereditary factors are very important in terms of susceptibility to SZ. Accumulating data from genome-wide association studies (GWAS) are constantly decoding SZ risk genes. Especially with the widespread use of new generation sequencing systems, it has been shown that more than 200 loci may play a role in the etiology. In addition, epigenetic factors should not be forgotten. Biomarker studies (Brain Derived Neurotrophic Factor (BDNF), MB-COMT, COMT, Reelin (RELN) and The serotonin receptor subtype 2 (HTR2) etc.) have proven that DNA methylation and histone acetylation are also effective in the development of SZ. The use of epigenetic treatments in practice and the development of gene therapy options provide hope for the treatment of such neuropsychiatric diseases. SZ is a severe mental-psychiatric disorder for which there is no definite knowledge about its underlying mechanisms. Although the complex interactions of genetic and environmental factors play a role in the etiology of SZ, studies on twins have shown that hereditary factors are very important in terms of susceptibility to SZ. Heritability is the proportion of variance, in a multifactorial threshold model, explained by genetic variability. The concordance rates of SZ for monozygotic twins have been found to be approximately %50–60, compared with %6–%10 in dizygotic twins. Additionally, studies have shown elevated rates of SZ and SZ spectrum disorders in biological families of schizophrenic adoptees compared with biological families of control adoptees, coupled with low, equivalent such rates in adoptive families of both types of adoptees (**Table 3**).

The consanguineous relationship seems to be valid not only for the disease but also for the inheritance of some brain morphology changes that may be related to the disease. In a neuroimaging study of families with multiple affected individuals, the brain structures of patients and unaffected relatives showed similar aberrations to their relatives with SZ, and the greater the degree of kinship, that is, the greater the genetic similarity, the more similar the degree of deviation was [76–78]. Considering all the information accumulated so far, it is known that SZ is familial and genes make the most important contribution to the risk of the disease. There are different chromosomal regions pointed out by linkage studies. Accumulating data from GWAS are constantly decoding SZ risk genes. Especially with the widespread use of new generation sequencing systems, it has been shown that more than 200 loci may play a role in the etiology. Copy Number Variations (CNVs) are stretches of genomic deletions and duplications ranging from 1 kb to several Mb, and thus are likely to have larger phenotypic effects than Single Nucletoide Polymorphisms (SNPs). A well-known CNV is the 22q11 deletion, 20–30% of people with it having SZ [79]. Additionally, There are many CNV Loci associated with SZ (**Table 4**) [80–82].

This study identified 108 independent genomic risk loci, localizing the search to genes that are current or promising targets for treatment (DRD2, GRM3, NOTCH4), genes more widely involved in glutamatergic neurotransmission (GRIN2A, SRR, CLCN3, and GRIA1), and unexpected candidate mechanisms involving neuronal calcium signaling (CACNA1C, CACNA1l, CACNB2, RIMS1) and broader synaptic function (KCTD13, CNTN4, PAK6). When considering all researches, studies have indicated that APOE, BDNF, CHRNA7, COMT, DISC1, DRD2, HTR2A, and NRG1 genes are as strong candidate genes in the etiology of SZ [83–85]. Considering all studies, it can be said that SZ is a multigenic, multifactorial neuropsychiatric disease.

Relation	Risk (%)
General population	0.86
Identical twins	57.70
First-degree relatives	
Brothers and Sisters	8.5
Children	8.2
Third-degree relatives (first cousin)	2.9
Risk of offspring of 0–2 schizophrenic parents	
Neither parents schizophrenic	8.2
One parent schizophrenic	13.8
Both parents schizophrenic	36.6

Table 3.
Risks to relatives of those with schizophrenia by Dr. Özdemir.

CNV Loci	Related gene(s)/syndromes
1q21.1 deletion/duplication	Connexin50, GJA8
2p16.3 deletion	NRXN1
3q29 deletion	PAK2, DLG1, FBXO45
7q36.3 duplication	VIPR2
15q13.2 deletion/duplication	Williams–Beuren Syndrome
16p13.11/16p11.2 duplication	—
17q12 deletion/duplication	Many genes
22q11.2 deletion	Di Geoge syndrome

Abbreviations: Connexin50, Gap Junction Protein Alpha 8 (GJA8), Neurexin 1 (NRXN1), The p21-activated kinase 2 (PAK2), Discs large homolog 1 (DLG1), F-Box Protein 45 (FBXO45), Vasoactive intestinal peptide receptor 2 (VIPR2), Copy Number Variations (CNVs). The Psychiatric Genomics Consortium (PGC) published the most extensive GWAS report on SZ in 2014 (up to 36,989 cases and 113,075 controls).

Table 4.
The most important CNV loci associated with schizophrenia by Özdemir.

Gene	DNA metilation status	Brain region
RELN	Hyper-methylation of promoter in SZ	Frontal/occipital lobe pre-frontal cortex
MB-COMT	Hypomethylation of MB-COMT promoter	DLPFC (Broadman's area46)
SOX10	Hyper-methylation of SOX10 in SZ	Prefrontal cortex (BA10)
FOXP2	Hyper-methylation of FOXP2 in SZ	Parahippocampus gyrus

Abbreviations: reelin (RELN), SRY-box transcription factor 10 (SOX10), Forkhead box protein P2 (FOXP2), schizophrenia (SZ).

Table 5.
Candidate genes in DNA methylation studies by Özdemir.

In addition, epigenetic factors should not be forgotten Changes in DNA methylation and other epigenetic factors (histone acetylation, miRNA, etc.) are thought to be more common and more effective than expected in the etiology of SZ. The advancement of next-generation sequencing technology has provided an opportunity for genome-wide methylation studies, termed epigenome-wide association studies (EWAS). DNA methylation changes in SZ have been explored using candidate genes strategy and whole genome approaches and some candidate genes given in **Table 5**.

Biomarker studies (BDNF, MB-COMT, COMT, RELN and HTR2 etc) have proven that DNA methylation and histone acetylation are also effective in the development of SZ. The use of epigenetic treatments in practice and the development of gene therapy options provide hope for the treatment of such neuropsychiatric diseases.

microRNAs (miRs) are small single-stranded non-coding RNA molecules that functions in RNA silencing and post-transcriptional regulation of gene expression. They are approximately 22 nucleotides of length and transcribed from different regions of the genome and believed to have a crucial role in the development of central nervous system reported that the upregulation of miR-132 in the mouse led to the downregulation of its target genes during brain development. it is found substantial correlation networks between miR-92a, miR-495, and miR-134, and their target genes [B-cell lymphoma/leukemia 11A (BCL11A), Proteolipid Protein 1

Upregulated miRNAs	Downregulated miRNAs
miR-21-5p, miR-22-3p, miR-30d-5p, miR-30e-5p, miR-34a, miR-92a-3p, miR-106b, miR-122, miR-130a, miR-130b, miR-137, miR-181b-5p, miR-195-5p, miR-193-a-3p, miR-193b, miR-502-3p, miR-652, miR-886-5p	miR-7, miR-9-3p, miR-20b, miR-24, miR-26b, miR-29a, miR-29b, miR-29c, miR-30a-5p, miR-30b, miR-30d, miR-30e, miR-92, miR-128, miR-132, miR-132-5p, miR-134, miR-181b, miR-195, miR-200c, miR-212, miR-664-5p, miR-1271, miR-432,

Abbrevations: microRNA (miR).

Table 6.
miRNA dysregulation in schizophrenia by Özdemir.

(PLP1), and Synaptotagmin 11 (SYT11)] in pathways involved in oligodendrocyte function and neurodevelopment. Apart from these miRNAs, many miRNAs were found to be associated with SZ and could be biomarkers in the diagnosis of SZ (see in **Table 6**) [86–90].

Technological advances in medical genetics (NGS, whole exome and genome sequence analysis) facilitate the identification of candidate genes and the determination of etiology in SZ and other neuropsychiatric diseases. Especially with studies in the fields of epigenetics (DNA methylation, histone modification, miRNA) and gene therapy, genetics will be effective not only in the diagnosis of these diseases but also in the treatment management.

6. In-silico applications in schizophrenia and future perspectives

Because of the variability of this mental condition and the lack of particular useful biomarkers, diagnosing SZ is a difficult task. A few clinical signs, including physical, psychiatric, and psychological markers, must be investigated to diagnose SZ [91–93]. Various diagnostics, such as blood testing and medical imaging, are included in clinical evaluations [93, 94]. If the doctors cannot uncover a physical cause for the patient's suspected SZ symptoms, they may refer them to a psychiatrist, psychologist, or another expert in the field. Clinical interviews based on the diagnostic and statistical manual (DSM-IV) of mental disorders undertaken by clinical psychiatrists to diagnose patients with SZ are the mainstay of psychological assessment [95, 96]. Another major group of procedures capable of diagnosing SZ is functional and structural neuroimaging techniques [97, 98]. Structural neuroimaging modalities primarily comprise structural magnetic resonance imaging (sMRI) [99–101] and diffusion tensor imaging (DTI) [102, 103], which, due to their high spatial resolution, display the anatomy of the human brain and its structural connectivity respectively. Overall, structural neuroimaging modalities based on MRI are useful for visualizing white matter (WM), gray matter (GM), and CSF tissues of the brain, as well as investigating their anomalies [104, 105].

Functional neuroimaging modalities for the diagnosis of SZ include electroencephalography (EEG) [106], magnetoencephalography (MEG) [107], functional near-infrared spectroscopy (fNIRS) [108, 109], and functional MRI (fMRI) [110, 111]. The use of MEG and fNIRS to diagnose SZ has been limited due to their high cost and lack of accuracy. Nowadays, computer-aided diagnosis systems (CADS) have been proposed to assist clinicians in diagnosing SZ automatically utilizing modern image processing and AI approaches [112–114]. To produce extremely accurate and robust CADS, researchers used traditional machine learning (ML) and deep learning (DL) techniques [115]. Machine learning (ML) and artificial intelligence have recently been used for the diagnosis, monitoring, and prognosis of a variety of disorders, including SZ since these approaches, perform well in detecting a link between disease symptoms and disease. The results of studies using magnetic resonance imaging data and physiological signals as input data are given. To anticipate and monitor SZ, ML is used to extract key characteristics. A wide number of research suggest that a support vector machine, deep neural network, and random forest can accurately predict SZ with a 70–90% accuracy. Finally, the findings suggest that machine learning technologies offer clinicians credible responses when making judgments concerning SZ patients. In the field of biological psychiatry, there is a rising interest in using AI and machine learning [116–119]. Researchers in machine learning and artificial intelligence (ML and AI) use mathematical models to extract attributes or features from signals and pictures to establish links between the characteristics and brain state to evaluate if the brain is normal [120]. Scientists are interested in ML because certain ML algorithms can identify nonlinear correlations among characteristics, making it a great tool for unraveling patterns in SZ datasets. These, in turn, can anticipate disorders like SZ and track the nonlinear character of a condition. Support vector machine (SVM), random forest (RF), Naive Bayes (NB), artificial neural network (ANN), logistic regression (LR), and deep neural network (DNN) approaches are examples of extremely accurate machine learning methods. A CNN architecture is demonstrated in **Figure 2**.

Machine learning (ML) may be used to create computer-assisted diagnostic tools for clinical usage and to investigate disease pathophysiology. By allowing researchers to tackle the tremendous complexity of EEG data, machine learning has changed the area of SZ. Traditional machine learning (non-deep learning (DL) algorithm) has been the method of choice in EEG analysis for the past few years. It's been mixed and matched using a variety of feature extraction techniques [121–122]. DL algorithms have been widely used in medical image and signal processing in recent advancements, indicating that they offer a lot of research potential. In the vast majority of circumstances, they outperform standard machine learning algorithms. Many researchers have utilized DL in the field of EEG to investigate mental health to diagnose and classify diseases [123–126].

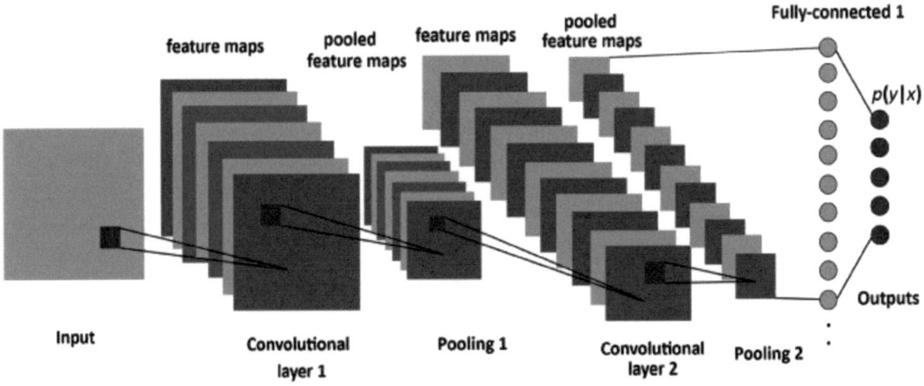

Figure 2.
A structure of a convolutional neural network by Dr. Ergüzel.

6.1 Entropy

EEG signals are studied utilizing changes in signal time series in time-domain feature extraction methods. The irregularity or unpredictability of brain activity is reflected in the EEG's complexity. Many researchers use nonlinear analytic methods to analyze EEG data as nonlinear theory continues to progress and evolve. Entropy is a nonlinear analytic technique for determining complexity. Entropy is the most widely used feature index among time-domain characteristics, and it is widely used in an illness diagnosis. Fuzzy entropy (FuzzyEn) is a regularly used entropy that was built based on other entropies. They have good resilience and high antinoise ability, and the algorithm complexity is lower than other entropies such as information entropy, sample entropy, and FuzzyEn. The entropy value measured by fuzzy entropy is continuously stable and less sensitive to the noise of EEG data, which makes it more suitable for analyzing chaotic signals. Previous studies have proven that the ability of FuzzyEn to detect and recognize signals is superior to the ability of other entropies for both epilepsy [36] and SZ [127]. The EEG signals of subjects with SZ were more random and, therefore, had a greater approximate entropy compared to the EEG signals of healthy subjects [128]. In addition, as previously reported using multiscale entropy, the complexity of schizophrenic patients is higher than that of the control group [129]. A broad overview Deep learning is the use of deep (multi-layer) artificial neural networks (DNNs), a class of problem-solving or system-modeling algorithms inspired by the nervous system that, unlike typical software, learn to solve issues through training [130]. DNNs have performed well in jobs that were previously regarded to be the only province of human competence. They have demonstrated exceptional performance in a variety of areas, including speech recognition [131], language translation [132], text understanding and generation [133], and object detection and recognition in images and videos [134].

DNNs are classed as feedforward or recurrent based on the direction of information flow. The information flow in feedforward DNNs is from input to output without any feedback loops (e.g., analogous to feedforward connections from V1 to V2 in the visual system). Feedforward multilayered DNNs are universal approximators, meaning that they can estimate with arbitrary precision any mapping (function) between inputs (e.g., pictures) and outputs (e.g., categories in a classification job) of a static system [135]. This type of DNN is most commonly utilized in activities that do not require any changes in time (e.g., image recognition). Recurrent DNNs, on the other hand, incorporate feedback loops in which layers communicate feedback information to each other and layers higher in the hierarchy.

Recurrent DNNs are universal approximators of dynamical systems, similar to feedforward DNNs [136]. This form of DNN is commonly employed in data that changes over time or is ordinal (e.g., weather forecasting or language translation). DNNs' ability to approximate complicated, multivariate, nonlinear systems vastly outperforms the results produced with classic shallow networks and machine learning methodologies, according to empirical studies. DNNs are end-to-end techniques, which means they not only learn to solve a job (e.g., speech recognition), but also automatically extract an optimal collection of features from the raw data that will be utilized to perform the problem. This is one of the reasons for their huge success in solving complex tasks.

DNNs can overcome various restrictions and biases influencing human-produced features by learning to extract features directly from raw data, resulting in improved performance with less task-specific customization. A DNN architecture that classifies animal species using raw photos as input, for example, can be taught to handle a wide range of different tasks, such as face recognition, cell type classification, or MRI-based disease detection, with no changes to the output/classification layer. Because DNNs must learn a large number of parameters to differentiate important from irrelevant information in the often high-dimensional and noisy input space, the benefits of autonomous extraction come at the cost of enormous training datasets. Despite recent breakthroughs in autonomous DNN design [137, 138], three critical components of DNN design continue to rely heavily on human judgment: 2) learning rules (training algorithm): techniques for changing network weights during training; 3) objective functions: performance or cost measurements linked with an output (e.g., error, reward) that DNNs learn to minimize or maximize during training [139]. Deep learning can be used to delineate the structural characteristics of schizophrenia and to provide supplementary diagnostic information in clinical settings.

In **Figure 3**, the number of papers evaluated by the ANN architecture. (b) The ANN architecture's stated accuracy in the binary diagnostic test. (c) Several peer-reviewed studies are organized by data modality. (d) The binary diagnostic task's stated accuracy per data modality. (e) ANN architecture and publication year for several peer-reviewed studies. (f) A comparison of the accuracy reported by research employing datasets from various data collection sites when models were assessed on data from training sites (pooled sites evaluation) versus data from held-out sites that were not utilized during training (held-out sites evaluation) (leave-one-site-out evaluation). The sample sizes (number of participants) of the studies are represented by the size of the circles in panels (b) and (d), and the orange circles emphasize the five studies indicated in panels (a) (f).

6.2 Metaverse

SZ is a severe mental disorder characterized by positive (hallucinations, delusions, muddled thinking, and disorganized speech) and negative (affective flatness, alogia, and avolition) symptoms, as well as language impairment [141]. Individuals with SZ have a higher risk of suicide; the lifetime rate of suicide in those with SZ is around 10% [142]. The most obvious possible consequence of virtual contact is on psychoses, particularly those involving delusions and/or hallucinations. These are not the only conceivable outcomes, nor are they the most prevalent, so we must be explicit about this. Overuse of digital technology is linked to a variety of mental health disorders, including somatic symptoms (6%), sadness (4%), psychoticism (0.5%), paranoid ideation (0.5%), and serious mental disease (2%). However, psychoses are among the most significant, and they demand considerable thought, especially if a firm with an estimated 1.9 billion daily users suggests a shift to a digitally immersive experience. Facebook's Reality Labs Division appears to be sketching out the design of their metaverse and how it would simulate interacting with people, much as in a game.

In connection with excessive use of digital technology, schizotypal personality characteristics such as odd experiences, impulsive nonconformity, and cognitive disorganization have garnered attention [143]. Schizotypy is thought to be a subclinical illness related to SZ. Due to the complications that studies with SZ might cause, evaluating schizotypy is frequently done instead of examining patients with SZ. In one research, 6100 20- to 30-year-olds were assessed for problematic internet usage (PIU), depression, anxiety, and schizotypal features. PIU was present in around 30% of these patients. In addition to the well-known connections between PIU, sadness, and anxiety, 2, PIU was linked to schizotypal personality features. Another study looked at the relationship between schizotypy symptoms, Facebook use, and PIU7. Two hundred

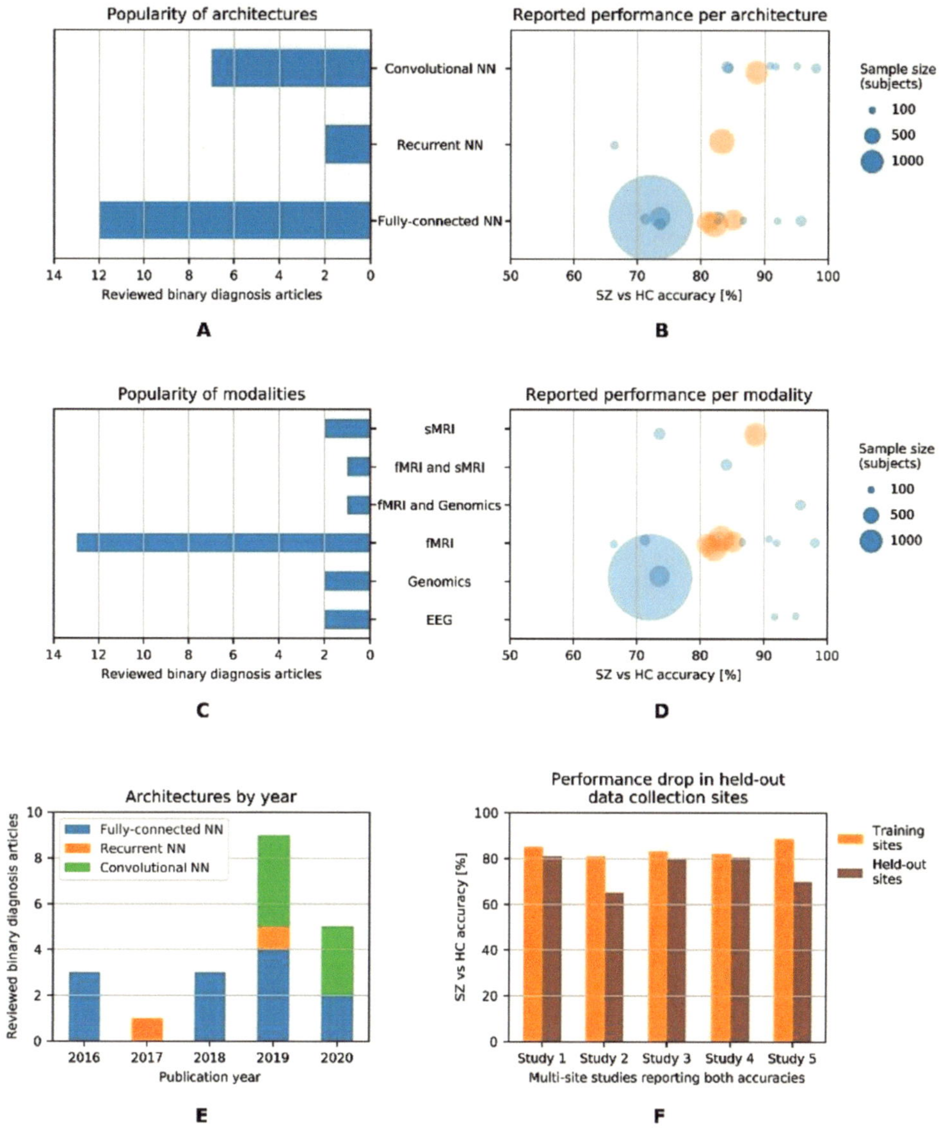

Figure 3.
Review of binary diagnosis of schizophrenic (SZ) patients against healthy controls (HC). (A) Number of reviewed articles by ANN architecture. (B) Reported accuracy of the binary diagnosis task by ANN architecture. (C) Number of reviewed articles by data modality. (D) Reported accuracy of the binary diagnosis task by data modality. (E) Number of reviewed articles by ANN architecture and publication year. (F) Comparison of the accuracy reported by studies using datasets from multiple data collection sites, when models were evaluated on data from collection sites used during training (pooled site evaluation) or on data from held-out sites that were not used during training (leave-one-site-out evaluation). In panels (B) and (D), the size of the circles represents the sample sizes (the number of subjects) of the studies, and the orange circles highlight the five studies showed on panel (F) [140].

seventy 18- to 30-year-olds took part in the study, and it was discovered that schizotypy levels predicted PIU as well as the frequency of Facebook use. PIU was better predicted by disorganized schizotypy. There is other research in this line, but the results are fairly consistent: There is a link between digital usage and schizotypy symptoms similar to SZ and other psychoses. Studies concentrating on subclinical symptoms related to schizotypy are thought to have minimal significance for clinically relevant diseases. Concerning digital usage, there are various professionally validated descriptions of SZ and psychoses. One clinical case series published in a recognized publication described two individuals who suffered Facebook-related delusions. " the backdrop of the nature of social networking media and the internet, including instances of how they have been utilized therapeutically, as well as the potential for negative usage," the authors said. While severe mental symptoms such as these are infrequent in PIU patients, around 0.5 percent report delusions and psychoses2. Even if 10% of the almost two billion daily Facebook users acquire PIU, it equates to around 1 million persons with psychosis or comparable symptoms who engage in virtual worlds regularly.

What can we draw from this research in the context of immersing a large number of social media users in a metaverse? At most, such an atmosphere may provide a temporary haven' for persons suffering from schizophrenic-like symptoms. It remains to be seen whether this makes the metaverse a safe place for other individuals. At worst, absorption in this digital environment may raise the probability of becoming disconnected from reality, resulting in delusional or psychotic symptoms. Once again, we are witnessing a situation in which a digital technology corporation proposes a product with a high potential for harm to public health that has not been subjected to adequate scientific risk assessment. It's unclear whether Facebook's investment in 10,000 employment in nations that have agreed to develop this technology has anything to do with it. The metaverse might become a psychotic sanctuary, feeding a certain form of sadism. It has the potential to send our society into a state of SZ, separating us from reality and transforming truth into a succession of delirious interpretations, ending in paranoia, delusions, and yet-unknown diseases in both realms. According to a new paper published in the journal The Lancet Psychiatry, researchers conducted the largest clinical trial employing VR therapy to treat individuals suffering from psychosis and SZ. The experiment was part of the game change program, created by the University of Oxford and the Oxford Health NHS Foundation Trust to treat agoraphobia, a typical symptom of psychosis [144].

7. Multimodal neuroimaging in schizophrenia

Multiple methods, and technologies that provide structural and functional data on neural mechanisms, including neuroimaging in general, electroencephalography (EEG), magnetoencephalography (MEG), functional magnetic resonance imaging (fMRI), positron emission (PET), diffusion tensor imaging (DTI) and noninvasive modalities. Although each modality provides different and valuable information about brain structures and/or activities, researchers have begun to combine multiple techniques called multimodal neuroimaging (MN) to understand brain dynamics in more detail and to overcome the limitations of modalities. Multimodal neuroimaging has several advantages over unimodal neuroimaging in providing more comprehensive information on quantifying, generalizing, and normalizing neural processes and structures, higher spatial and temporal resolution, and it has been shown to reduce the limitations of unimodal techniques. Multimodal neuroimaging; is thought to have the potential to shed light on the neuronal mechanisms underlying risky conditions such as structural and functional pathophysiological features, prefronto-temporal gray matter reduction, and impaired high-grade cognitive processing, and impaired dopaminergic-glutamatergic neurotransmission in schizophrenia patients [145]. Recent advances in machine learning techniques have allowed promising results for personalized prediction and characterization in patients with schizophrenia [146]. In studies combining DTI and rest or task fMRI; DTI and task fMRI analyses revealed fractional anisotropy (FA) reductions in the right medial temporal lobe adjacent to the right parahippocampal gyrus, and fMRI was reported to reveal partial hypoactivation of prefrontal, superior parietal, and occipital in patients with schizophrenia [147]. DTI and fMRI at rest showed altered functional and anatomical connectivity in the medial frontal and anterior cingulate gyrus in patients with schizophrenia [148]. In the DTI and on-the-job fMRI study, it was reported that significantly reduced activation of the fronto-striato-cingulate network in patients with schizophrenia was associated with difficulties in making decisions under uncertainty. The same study shows that activation in parts of the fronto-striato-cingulate network is negatively correlated with an increased radial spread in temporal white matter [149]. Another similar study showed that the total connectivity of the thalamus to the lateral frontal cortex (LPFC) is reduced in patients with schizophrenia. Total thalamocortical connectivity to the LPFC predicts working memory performance and also correlated with LPFC BOLD activation. The correlation with BOLD activation of the LPFC is emphasized in patients with schizophrenia [150]. A proposed new framework for the classification of schizophrenic patients and healthy control subjects based on using both fMRI and band-limited envelope correlation measures in MEG to interrogate functional network components at rest provides evidence that the combination of these two methods is useful for estimating patients with schizophrenia. The results suggest that the combination of these two methods provides valuable information that captures key features of brain network connectivity in schizophrenia. Independent component analysis (ICA)-based functional network connectivity (FNC) is a data-driven approach that summarizes the overall link between individual brain maps over time. Therefore, the FNC feature provides a picture of the connectivity pattern over time between individual components. The blood oxygenation level-dependent (BOLD) response as measured by fMRI, while allowing high spatial resolution maps, is limited because it is an indirect and slow physiological signal. Neural oscillatory activity, including rhythmic electrical activity in cell ensembles, is thought to underlie BOLD responses. This neural oscillatory activity occurs in the ~1–900 Hz band; such fast electrical signals can only be measured directly with techniques such as MEG, rather than fMRI. Measuring resting-state brain activity in a common subject sample using both fMRI and MEG combines the strengths of each modality, allowing the comparison of hemodynamic and electrophysiological effects. In this way, it provides important information about FNC, which is of particular importance for the study of schizophrenia and similar conditions. Recent studies show that connection dynamics can capture repetitive patterns of interaction between internal networks during undetectable rest or task-related experiments with FNC. These repetitive interaction patterns contain valuable information for the individual prediction of patients with schizophrenia [151]. Numerous studies combining fMRI data and MEG data consistently show auditory-sensory processing deficits in patients with schizophrenia. Poor sensory gating has been characterized not only as a deficit in selective attention and/or the formation of memory traces, but also as a useful biomarker of cognitive and social dysfunction observed in patients with schizophrenia. Electroencephalographic (EEG) and MEG studies of sensory gating implicate the temporal lobes, including the superior temporal gyrus, as the most likely neuronal producer of the sensory gating deficit. Hippocampal hypoactivation, which can be demonstrated by invasive methods in weak sensory gating, could be demonstrated by combining EEG, MEG and fMRI findings. Impaired sensory gating is thought to be an endophenotypic marker for schizophrenia. When the neural mechanisms underlying the multi-sensory integration of auditory and visual stimuli in schizophrenia patients and healthy controls were examined using MEG and fMRI together with structural MRI (sMRI), it was shown that patients with schizophrenia had slower reaction times to multisensory stimuli than healthy controls. Because associated areas of the temporal lobe are essential for the integration of auditory and visual information, altered multisensory processing is consistent with the findings that patients with schizophrenia show functional and anatomical differences in the temporal lobes. The long-term goal is to identify local cortical deficiencies as well as deficiencies in cortical networks that lead to the abnormalities observed in patients with schizophrenia. Knowledge about these deficiencies, assessment of associations with neurochemical abnormalities, and ultimately, may lead to more individually targeted pharmacological interventions. The prefrontal cortex (PFC) and hippocampal structures play a central role in working memory and relational memory disorders exhibited in patients with schizophrenia. PFC and hippocampal functional deficiencies have traditionally been attributed to the characteristics of cortical structures. However, according to an alternative view, it has been reported that there is a functional disconnection between the frontal and temporal cortices (). In a study to demonstrate this, 3 T MRI was used [8]. Functional (ie, fMRI, PET) and biochemical/structural (ie, 1H-MRS, DTI, voxel-based morphometry (VBM). It is not possible to determine whether the disease underlies core deficits or represents compensation for overcoming primary functional deficits. However, MEG results suggest hypersynchronous prefrontal and temporal networks are thought to be consistent with the disconnected model of schizophrenia [98].

8. Conclusion

Over the last two decades, several trends have collided to raise questions about how the notions of schizophrenia, the schizophrenia spectrum, and the psychotic disorders spectrum should be viewed. These tendencies can be found in fields including genetics, neuroimaging, and data-driven computational investigations of numerous response systems. Growing evidence reveals that schizophrenia is a broad and heterogeneous condition that is part of a multi-faceted psychosis spectrum, rather than a single disease entity. The reliance on sets of symptoms and signs for defining a diagnosis, as well as the use of traditional diagnostic categories in analyzing clinical research grants, has slowed progress in explaining these varied developments. In order to address these issues this chapters covered the topic from different perspectives. The chapter takes a neurological approach to schizophrenia and discusses individualized treatment options from diverse perspectives. Genotyping and phenotyping keys are used to provide personalized treatment in the diagnosis and treatment of schizophrenia. The psychopharmacology of schizophrenia and the mechanism of action of antipsychotic medicines are discussed after comorbid schizophrenia in addiction with the use of numerous substances. In the last section, in-silico application and computational methodologies encompassing feature extraction process and destructive impact of metaverse are shared. Recent studies underline the success and contribution to biomarker extraction process of collaborative studies.

Conflict of interest

The authors declare no conflict of interest.

Author details

Nevzat Tarhan[1*], Nesrin Dilbaz[1], Bahruz Shukurov[2], Ceylan Ergul[1], Guner Ulak[1], Yesim Ozdemir[1], Turker Tekin Erguzel[1] and Firdevs Seyfe Sen[1]

1 Uskudar University, Istanbul, Turkey

2 NP Istanbul Brain Hospital, İstanbul, Turkey

*Address all correspondence to: nevzat.tarhan@uskudar.edu.tr

References

[1] Hiemke C, Bergemann N, Clement HW, Conca A, Deckert J, Domschke K, et al. Consensus guidelines for therapeutic drug monitoring in neuropsychopharmacology: Update 2017. Pharmacopsychiatry. 2018;**51**:9-62. DOI: 10.1055/s-0043-116492. DOI: 10.1055/s-0043-116492

[2] Axelrod J, Tomchick R. Enzymatic o-methylation of epinephrine and other catechols. The Journal of Biological Chemistry. 1958;**233**:702-705. DOI: 10.1016/ S0021-9258(18)64731-3

[3] Weinshilboum R, Raymond F. Variations in catechol-O-methyltransferase activity in inbred strains of rats. Neuropharmacology. 1977;**16**:703-706. DOI: 10.1016/ 0028-3908(77)90124-1

[4] Chen J, Lipska BK, Halim N, Ma QD, Matsumoto M, Melhem S, et al. Functional analysis of genetic variation in catechol-O-methyltransferase (COMT): Effects on mRNA, protein, and enzyme activity in postmortem human brain. American Journal of Human Genetics. 2004;**75**:807-821. DOI: 10.1086/425589

[5] Canbolat F, Dilek M, Sercan C, Tarhan N, Rgier eD, Farmer M, Rae D, et al. Evaluating of solute carrier family 6 member 4 gene (SLC6A4) promoter polymorphisms with escitalopram plasma levels for precision medicine in major depressive disorder. The Journal of Neurobehavioral Sciences. 2021;8(1): 62-69. DOI:10.4103/jnbs. jnbs_44_20

[6] Canbolat F, Dilek M, Evrensel A, Aydın A, Tarhan N. Quantitation of escitalopram and its metabolites by liquid chromatography-tandem mass spectrometry in psychiatric patients: New metabolic ratio establishment. Basic & Clinical Pharmacology & Toxicology. 2018;**124**:285-297. DOI: 10.1111/ bcpt.13133

[7] Mrazek D. Psychiatric Pharmacogenomics. Oxford University Press; 2010 ISBN-13: 9780195367294

[8] Boileau I, Assaad JM, Pihl RO, et al. Alcohol promotes dopamine release in the human nucleus accumbens. Synapse. 2003;**49**:226-231. DOI: 10.1002/syn.10226

[9] Martins SS, Gorelick DA. Conditional substance abuse and dependence by diagnosis of mood or anxiety disorder or schizophrenia in the U.S. population. Drug and Alcohol Dependence. 2011;**119**:28-36. DOI: 10.1016/j. drugalcdep.2011.05.010

[10] Green AI, Noordsy DL, Brunette MF, et al. Substance abuse and schizophrenia: pharmacotherapeutic intervention. Journal of Substance Abuse Treatment. 2008;**34**(1):61-71. DOI: 10.1016/j. jsat.2007.01.008

[11] Turkington A, Mulholland CC, Rushe TM, et al. Impact of persistent substance misuse on 1-year outcome in first-episode psychosis. The British Journal of Psychiatry. 2009;**195**(3):242-248. DOI: 10.1192/bjp.bp.108.057471

[12] Dilbaz N, Göğcegöz I, Noyan CO. Kazan Kızılkurt, Bağımlılık Tanı ve Tedavi Temel Kitabı. Ankara: Nobel Tıp Kitapevleri; 2021 ISBN: 9786257146777

[13] Ereshefsky L, Jann MW, Saklad SR, Davis CM, Richards AL, Burch NR. Effects of smoking on fluphenazine clearance in psychiatric inpatients. Biological Psychiatry. 1985;**20**:329-332. DOI: 10.1016/0006-3223(85)90063-0

[14] Jann MW, Saklad SR, Ereshefsky L, Richards AL, Harrington CA, Davis CM. Effects of smoking on haloperidol and reduced haloperidol plasma concentrations and haloperidol clearance. Psychopharmacology. 1986;**90**:468-470. DOI: 10.1007/BF00174062

[15] Bozikas VP, Papakosta M, Niopas I, Karavatos A, Mirtsou-Fidani V. Smoking impact on CYP1A2 activity in a group of patients with schizophrenia. European Neuropsychopharmacology. 2004;**14**:39-44. DOI: 10.1016/s0924-977x(03)00061-0

[16] Schneier FR, Siris SG. A review of psychoactive substance use and abuse in schizophrenia: Patterns of drug choice. The Journal of Nervous and Mental Disease. 1987;**175**(641-652):21. DOI: 10.1097/00005053-198711000-00001

[17] Barnes TR, Mutsatsa SH, Hutton SB, Watt HC, Joyce EM. Comorbid substance use and age at onset of schizophrenia. The British Journal of Psychiatry. 2006;**188**:237-242. DOI: 10.1192/bjp.bp.104.007237

[18] Green B, Young R, Kavanagh D. Cannabis use and misuse prevalence among people with psychosis. British Journal of Psychiatry. 2005;**187**:306-313. DOI: 10.1192/bjp.187.4.306

[19] Andreasson S, Allebeck P, Engstrom A, Rydberg U. Cannabis and schizophrenia. A longitudinal study of Swedish conscripts. Lancet. 1987;**26**(2):1483-1486. DOI: 10.1016/s0140-6736(87)92620-1

[20] Dean B, Sundram S, Bradbury R, Scarr E, Copolov D. Studies on (3H) CP-55940 binding in the human central nervous system; regional spesific changes in dansity of cannabinoid-1 receptors associated with schizophrenia and cannabis use. Neuroscience. 2001;**103**:9-15. DOI: 10.1016/s0306-4522(00)00552-2

[21] Caspi A, Moffitt TE, Cannon M, McClay J, Murray R, Harrington H, et al. Moderation of the effect of adolescent-onset cannabis use on adult psychosis by a functional polymorphism in the catechol-O methyltransferase gene: Longitudinal evidence of a gene X environment interaction. Biological Psychiatry. 2005;**57**:1117-1127. DOI: 10.1016/j.biopsych.2005.01.026

[22] Dixon L, Haas G, Weiden PJ, Sweeney J, Frances AJ. Drug abuse in schizophrenic patients: clinical correlates and reasons for use. The American Journal of Psychiatry. 1991;**148**:224-230. DOI: 10.1176/ajp.148.2.224

[23] Buckley PF. Substance abuse in schizophrenia: A review. The Journal of Clinical Psychiatry. 1998;**59**(26-30):26

[24] Dankı D, Dilbaz N, Okay T, et al. Madde kullanımına Bağlı Gelişen Psikotik Bozuklukta Atipik Antipsikotik Tedavisi: Bir Gözden Geçirme. Bağımlılık Dergisi. 2005;**6**:136-141. DOI: 10.26650/experimed.2020.0005

[25] Niemi-Pynttäri JA, Sund R, Putkonen H, et al. Substance-induced psychoses converting into schizophrenia: A register-based study of 18,478 Finnish inpatient cases. The Journal of Clinical Psychiatry. 2013;**74**(1):94-99. DOI: 10.4088/JCP.12m07822

[26] Grant KM, LeVan TD, Wells SM, et al. Methamphetamine-associated psychosis. Journal of Neuroimmune Pharmacology. 2012;**7**(1):113-139. DOI: 10.1007/s11481-011-9288-1

[27] Van Dorn RA, Desmarais SL, Scott Young M, et al. Assessing illicit drug use among adults with schizophrenia.

Psychiatry Research. 2012;**200**:228-236. DOI: 10.1016/j.psychres.2012.05.028

[28] Brizer DA, Hartman N, Sweeney J, et al. Effect of methadone plus neuroleptics on treatment-resistant chronic paranoid schizophrenia. The American Journal of Psychiatry. 1985;**142**(9):1106-1107. DOI: 10.1176/ajp.142.9.1106

[29] Sullivan MD, Edlund MJ, Zhang L, et al. Association between mental health disorders, problem drug use, and regular prescription opioid use. Archives of Internal Medicine. 2006;**166**:2087-2093. DOI: 10.1001/archinte.166.19.2087

[30] Pullen GP, Best NR, Maguire J. Anticholinergic drug abuse: A common problem? British Medical Journal (Clinical Research Ed.). 1984;**289**:612-613. DOI: 10.1136/bmj.289.6445.612

[31] Tandon R, Greden JF. Cholinergic hyperactivity and negative schizophrenic symptoms. A model of cholinergic/dopaminergic interactions in schizophrenia. Archives of General Psychiatry. 1989;**46**(8):745-753. DOI: 10.1001/archpsyc.1989.01810080075010

[32] Warner R, Taylor D, Wright J, et al. Substance use among the mentally ill: Prevalence, reasons for use, and effects on illness. American Journal of Orthopsychiatry. 1994;**64**(1):30-39. DOI: 10.1037/h0079489

[33] Dilbaz N, Darçın AE. Şizofreni ve madde kullanım bozukluğu eş tanılı hastalarda tedavi. Klinik Psikofarmakol Bulteni. 2011;**21**(1):80-90. DOI: 10.5350/KPB-BCP201121114

[34] Soyka M. Dual diagnosis in patients with schizophrenia. Issues in Pharmacological Treatment. CNS Drugs. 1996;**5**(414-25):48. DOI: 10.2165/00023210-199605060-00002

[35] Wobrock T, Pajonk FG, D' Amelio R, Falkai P. Schizophrenia and addiction. Psychoneuro. 2005;**31**(9):433-440. DOI: 10.1007/s00406-006-0707-x

[36] McEvoy JP, Freudenreich O, Levin ED, Rose JE. Haloperidol increases smoking in patients with schizophrenia. Psychopharmacology. 1995;**119**:124-126. DOI: 10.1007/BF02246063

[37] Yovell Y, Opler LA. Clozapine reverses cocaine craving in a treatment-resistant mentally ill chemical abusers: case report and hypothesis. The Journal of Nervous and Mental Disease. 1994;**182**(10):591-592. DOI: 10.1097/00005053-199410000-00017

[38] Buckley P, Thompson P, Way L, Meltzer HY. Substance abuse among patients with treatment resistant schizophrenia: Characteristics and implications for clozapine therapy. The American Journal of Psychiatry. 1994;**151**(385-9):67. DOI: 10.1176/ajp.151.3.385

[39] Albanese MJ, Khantzian EJ, Murphy SL, Green AI. Decreased substance use in chronically psychotic patients treated with clozapine. The American Journal of Psychiatry. 1994;**151**:780-781. DOI: 10.1176/ajp.151.5.780b

[40] Marcus P, Snyder R. Reduction of comorbid substance abuse with clozapin (letter). The American Journal of Psychiatry. 1995;**152**(959):70. DOI: 10.1176/ajp.152.6.959a

[41] Zimmet SV, Strous RD, Burgess ES, Kohnstamm S, Green AI. Effects of clozapine on substance use in patients with schizophrenia and schizoaffective disorder: A retrospective survey. Journal of Clinical Psychopharmacology. 1991;**2000**(20):94-98. DOI: 10.1097/00004714-200002000-00016

[42] Kaya H, Dilbaz N, Okay T, Çeşmeci U. Ketiapin bağımlılık yapıyor mu? Klinik Psikofarmakoloji Bülteni. 2009;**19(Ek**:1):32-36

[43] Williams JM, Steinberg ML, Zimmermann MH, et al. Comparison of two intensities of tobacco dependence counseling in schizophrenia and schizoaffective disorder. Journal of Substance Abuse Treatment. 2010;**38**:384-393. DOI: 10.1016/j.jsat.2010.03.006

[44] George TP, Sernyak MJ, Ziedonis DM, Woods SW. Effects of clozapine on smoking in chronic schizophrenic outpatients. The Journal of Clinical Psychiatry. 1995;**56**:344-346

[45] de Leon J. Psychopharmacology: atypical antipsychotic dosing: The effect of smoking and caffeine. Psychiatric Services. 2004;**55**(5):491-493. DOI: 10.1176/appi.ps.55.5.491

[46] Potvin S, Blanchet P, Stip E. Substance abuse is associated with increased extrapyramidal symptoms in schizophrenia: A meta-analysis. Schizophrenia Research. 2009;**113**(2-3):181-188. DOI: 10.1016/j.schres.2009.06.010

[47] Galletly C, Castle D, Dark F, et al. Royal Australian and New Zealand College of Psychiatrists clinical practice guidelines for the management of schizophrenia and related disorders. The Australian and New Zealand Journal of Psychiatry. 2016;**50**(5):410-472. DOI: 10.1177/0004867416641195

[48] Jones PB, Buckley PF. Schizophrenia. UK: Elsevier; 2006 ISBN 0443 102503

[49] Kapur S, Seeman P. Does fast dissociation from the dopamine D2 receptor explain the action of atypical antipsychotics? A new hypothesis. Am J Psychiatry. 2001;**158**:360-369. DOI: 10.1176/appi.ajp.158.3.360

[50] Stahl S. Essential Psychopharmacology. 2nd ed. New York: Cambridge University Press; 2000. DOI: 10.2989/17280583.2014.914944

[51] Miyamoto S, Miyake N, Jarskog LF, et al. Pharmacological treatment of schizophrenia: A critical review of the pharmacology and clinical effects of current and future therapeutic agents. Molecular Psychiatry. 2012;**17**:1206-1227. DOI: 10.1038/mp.2012.47

[52] Laruelle M. Schizophrenia: From dopaminergic to glutamatergic interventions. Current Opinion in Pharmacology. 2014;**14**:97-102. DOI: 10.1016/j.coph.2014.01.001

[53] Seeman P. Dopamine receptor sequences. Therapeutic levels of neuroleptics occupy D2 receptors, clozapine occupies D4. Neuropsychopharmacology. 1992;7:261-284. DOI: 10.1021/cn400189s

[54] Miyamoto S, Duncan GE, Marx CE, Lieberman JA. Treatments for schizophrenia: A critical review of pharmacology and mechanisms of action of antipsychotic drugs. Molecular Psychiatry. 2005;**10**:79-104. DOI: 10.1038/sj.mp.4001556

[55] Stahl S. Key issues and unmet needs in schizophrenia. In: Kapur S, Lecrubier Y, editors. Dopamine in the Pathophysiology and Treatment of Schizophrenia. 2nd ed. London: Taylor & Francis; 2005. pp. 177-205. ISBN 1 84184 366 0. DOI: 10.3109/9780203427347-13

[56] Kapur S. Modulation of D2 receptors as a basis of antipsychotic effect. In: Kapur S, Lecrubier Y (2nd ed). Dopamine in the Pathophysiology and Treatment of Schizophrenia. Taylor & Francis; 2005. p:49-67 ISBN 1 84184 366 0. DOI: 10.3109/9780203427347-4

[57] Stahl SM. Stahl's Essential Psychopharmacology Neuroscientific Basis and Practical Application. Fourth Edition 2013. Cambridge University Press ISBN 978-1-107-02598-1 Hardback. DOI: 10.4103/0973-1229.58825

[58] Meltzer H. Multiple neurotransmitters involved in antipsychotic drug action. In: Kapur S, Lecrubier Y, editors. Dopamine in the Pathophysiology and Treatment of Schizophrenia. 2nd ed. London: CRC Press; 2003. pp. 177-205. ISBN 97804292211940. DOI: 10.3109/9780203427347

[59] Meltzer HY. Clinical studies on the mechanism of action of clozapine:the dopamine-serotonin hypothesis of schizophrenia. Psychopharmacology. 1989;**99**(Suppl):S18-S27. DOI: 10.1007/BF00442554

[60] Gray JA. Roth BL molecular targets for treating cognitive dysfunction in schizophrenia. Schizophrenia Bulletin. 2007;**33**:1100-1119. DOI: 10.1093/schbul/sbm074

[61] Barch DM. Pharmacological strategies for enhancing cognition in schizophrenia. Current Topics in Behavioral Neurosciences. 2010;**4**:43-96. DOI: 10.1007/7854_2010_39

[62] Stepnicki P, Kondej M, Kaczor AA. Current concepts and treatments of schizophrenia. Molecules. 2018;**23**:2087. DOI: 10.3390/molecules23082087

[63] Roth BL, Hanizavareh SM, Blum AE. Serotonin receptors represent highly favorable molecular targets for cognitive enhancement in schizophrenia and other disorders. Psychopharmacology. 2004;**174**:17-24. DOI: 10.1007/s00213-003-1683-8

[64] King MV, Marsden CA, Fone KC. A role for the 5-HT1A, 5-HT4 and 5-HT6 receptors in learning and memory. Trends in Pharmacological Sciences. 2008;**29**:482-492. DOI: 10.1016/j.tips.2008.07.001

[65] Carlsson A, Waters N, Holm-Waters S, et al. Interactions between monoamines, glutamate, and GABA in schizophrenia: New evidence. Annual Review of Pharmacology and Toxicology. 2001;**41**:237-260. DOI: 10.1146/annurev.pharmtox.41.1.237

[66] Yang AC, Tsai SJ. New Targets for schizophrenia treatment beyond the dopamine hypothesis. International Journal of Molecular Sciences. 2017;**18**(8):1689. DOI: 10.3390/ijms18081689

[67] Matosin N, Fernandez-Enright F, Frank E, et al. Metabotropic glutamate receptor mGluR2/3 and mGluR5 binding in the anterior cingulate cortex in psychotic and nonpsychotic depression, bipolar disorder and schizophrenia: Implications for novel mGluR-based therapeutics. J Psychiatry Neurosci JPN. 2014;**39**:407-416. DOI: 10.1503/JPN.130242

[68] Ward SE, Pennicott LE, Beswick P. AMPA receptor-positive allosteric modulators for the treatment of schizophrenia: An overview of recent patent applications. Future Medicinal Chemistry. 2015;**7**:473-491. DOI: 10.4155/fmc.15.4

[69] Javitt DC. Glycine transport inhibitors and the treatment of schizophrenia. Biological Psychiatry. 2008;**63**(1):6-8. DOI: 10.2174/1874104501004010010

[70] Rogóż Z, Kamińska K, Lech MA, Lorenc-Koci E. N-Acetylcysteine and aripiprazole improve social behavior and cognition and modulate brain BDNF levels in a rat model of schizophrenia. International Journal of Molecular

Sciences. 2022;**23**:2125. DOI: 10.3390/ijms23042125

[71] Bymaster FP, Felder C, Ahmed S, McKinzie D. Muscarinic receptors as a target for drugs treating schizophrenia. Current Drug Targets. CNS and Neurological Disorders. 2002;**1**(2):163-181. DOI: 10.2174/1568007024606249

[72] Ellenbroek BA, Ghiabi B. Do histamine receptor 3 antagonists have a place in the therapy for schizophrenia? Current Pharmaceutical Design. 2015;**21**:3760-3770. DOI: 10.2174/1381612821666150605105325

[73] Newman-Tancredi A, KlevenMS. Pharmacology of "atypicality" of antipsychotic drugs: Status and perspectives. Archives of Psychiatry and Psychotherapy. 2010;**4**:5-11

[74] Duinen MV, Reneerkens OAH, Lambrecht L, et al. Treatment of cognitive impairment in schizophrenia: Potential value of phosphodiesterase inhibitors in prefrontal dysfunction. Current Pharmaceutical Design. 2015;**21**:3813-3828. DOI: 10.2174/1381612821666150605110941

[75] Correll CU, Martin A, Charmi Patel C, et al. Systematic literature review of schizophrenia clinical practice guidelines on acute and maintenance management with antipsychotics. Schizophrenia. 2022;**8**:5. DOI: 10.1038/s41537-021-00192-x

[76] Henriksen Mads G, Nordgaar J, Jansson LB. Genetics of schizophrenia: Overview of methods, findings and limitations. Frontiers in Human Neuroscience. 2017;**11**:1-9. DOI: 10.3389/fnhum.2017.00322

[77] Gejman PV, Sanders AR, Kendler KS. Genetics of schizophrenia: New findings and challenges. Annual Review of Genomics and Human Genetics. 2011;**12**:121-144. DOI: 10.1146/annurev-genom-082410-101459

[78] Salleh MR. The Genetics of schizophrenia. MJMS. 2004;**11-2**:3-11

[79] Kotlar AV, Mercer KB, Mulle JG. New discoveries in schizophrenia genetics reveal neurobiological pathways: A review of recent findings. European Journal of Medical Genetics. 2015;**58**(12):704-714. DOI: 10.1016/j.ejmg.2015.10.008

[80] Chen CH, Cheng MC, Hu TM, Ping LT. Chromosomal microarray analysis as first-tier genetic test for schizophrenia. Front Gen. 2021;**12**:1-11. DOI: 10.3389/fgene.2021.620496

[81] Triful SC, Kohn B, Vlasie A. Bogdan-eduard patrıchı. Genetics of schizophrenia. Exp Ther Med. 2020;**20**:3462-3468. DOI: 10.3892/etm.2020.8973

[82] Reesl E, O'Donovan C, M, Owen MJ. Genetics of schizophrenia. Curr Opin Behavioral Science. 2015;**2**:8-14. DOI: 10.1016/j.cobeha.2014.07.001

[83] Foleyl C, Corvin A, Nakagome S. Genetics of schizophrenia: Ready to translate? Current Psychiatry Reports. 2017;**19**:61. DOI: 10.1007/s11920-017-0807-5

[84] Farrel MS, Werge T, Sklar P, Owen MJ, Ophoff RA, O'Donovan MC, et al. Evaluating historical candidate genes for schizophrenia. Molecular Psychiatry. 2015;**20**(5):555-562. DOI: 10.1038/mp.2015.16. DOI: 10.1038/mp.2015.16

[85] Rujescu D. Search for risk genes in schizophrenia. Der Nervenarzt. 2017;**88**(7):751-754. DOI: 10.1007/s00115-017-0330-2

[86] Khavari B, Cairns MJ. Epigenomic dysregulation in schizophrenia: In search of disease etiology and biomarkers. Cell. 2020;**9**:1837. DOI: 10.3390/cells9081837

[87] Rajman M, Schratt G. MicroRNAs in neural development: From master regulators to fine-tuners. Development. 2017;**144**:2310-2322. DOI: 10.1242/dev.144337

[88] Santarelli DM, Carroll AP, Cairns HM, Tooney PA, Cairns M.J. Schizophrenia-associated MicroRNA-gene interactions in the dorsolateral prefrontal cortex. Genom. Proteomics Bioinf. 2019;**17**:623-634. DOI: 10.1016/j.gpb.2019.10.003

[89] Shorter KR, Miller BH. Epigenetic mechanisms in schizophrenia. Progress in Biophysics and Molecular Biology. 2015;**118**(1-2):1-7. DOI: 10.1016/j.pbiomolbio.2015.04.008

[90] Heinrichs DW, Buchanan RW. Significance and meaning of neurological signs in schizophrenia. The American Journal of Psychiatry. 1998;**145**(1):11-18. DOI: 10.1176/ajp.145.1.11

[91] Boks MP, Russo S, Knegtering R, van den Bosch RJ. The specificity of neurological signs in schizophrenia: A review. Schizophrenia Research. 2000;**43**:109-116. DOI: 10.1016/S0920-9964(99)00145-0

[92] Wee ZY, Yong SWL, Chew QH, Guan C, Lee TS, Sim K. Actigraphy studies and clinical and biobehavioural correlates in schizophrenia: A systematic review. Journal of Neural Transmission. 2019;**126**:531-558. DOI: 10.1007/s00702-019-01993-2

[93] Tomasik J, Schwarz E, Guest PC, Bahn S. Blood test for schizophrenia. European Archives of Psychiatry and Clinical Neuroscience. 2012;**262**:79-83. DOI: 10.1007/s00406-012-0354-3

[94] Shenton ME, Kikinis R, Jolesz FA, et al. Abnormalities of the left temporal lobe and thought disorder in schizophrenia: A quantitative magnetic resonance imaging study. New England Journal of Medicine. 1992;**327**:604-612. DOI: 10.1056/NEJM199208273270905

[95] Siris SG. Diagnosis of secondary depression in schizophrenia: Implications for dsm-iv. Schizophrenia Bulletin. 1991;**17**:75-98. DOI: 10.1093/schbul/17.1.75

[96] Maj M. Critique of the DSM–IV operational diagnostic criteria for schizophrenia. The British Journal of Psychiatry. 1998;**172**:458-460. DOI: 10.1192/bjp.172.6.458

[97] McGuire P, Howes OD, Stone J, Fusar-Poli P. Functional neuroimaging in schizophrenia: diagnosis and drug discovery. Trends in Pharmacological Sciences. 2008;**29**:91-98. DOI: 10.1016/j.tips.2007.11.005

[98] Aine C, Bockholt HJ, Bustillo JR, et al. Multimodal neuroimaging in schizophrenia: Description and dissemination. Neuroinformatics. 2017;**15**:343-364. DOI: 10.1007/s12021-017-9338-9

[99] Sim K, DeWitt I, Ditman T, et al. Hippocampal and parahippocampal volumes in schizophrenia: A structural mri study. Schizophrenia Bulletin. 2006;**32**:332-340. DOI: 10.1093/schbul/sbj030

[100] Shenton ME, Dickey CC, Frumin M, McCarley RW. A review of MRI findings in schizophrenia. Schizophrenia Research. 2001;**49**:1-52. DOI: 10.1016/S0920-9964(01)00163-3

[101] Wisco JJ, Kuperberg GG, Manoach D, et al. Abnormal cortical folding patterns within broca's area

in schizophrenia: Evidence from structural mri. Schizophrenia Research. 2007;**94**:317-327. DOI: 10.1016/j.schres.2007.03.031

[102] Kyriakopoulos M, Bargiotas T, Barker GJ, Frangou S. Diffusion tensor imaging in schizophrenia. European Psychiatry. 2008;**23**:255-273. DOI: 10.1016/j.eurpsy.2007.12.004

[103] Kubicki M, McCarley R, Westin CF, Park HJ, Maier S, Kikinis R. A review of diffusion tensor imaging studies in schizophrenia. Journal of Psychiatric Research. 2007;**41**:15-30. DOI: 10.1016/j.jpsychires.2005.05.005

[104] Diwadkar VA, Pruitt P, Goradia D, et al. Fronto-parietal hypoactivation during working memory independent of structural abnormalities: conjoint FMRI and SMRI analyses in adolescent offspring of schizophrenia patients. NeuroImage. 2011;**58**:234-241. DOI: 10.1016/j. neuroimage.2011.06.033

[105] Varshney A, Prakash C, Mittal N, Singh P. A multimodel approach for schizophrenia diagnosis using FMRI and SMRI dataset. In: The International Symposium on Intelligent Systems Technologies and Applications. Vol. 530. Springer; 2016. pp. 869-877. DOI: 10.1007/978-3-319-47952-1_69

[106] Oh SL, Vicnesh J, Ciaccio EJ, Yuvaraj R, Acharya UR. Deep convolutional neural network model for automated diagnosis of schizophrenia using eeg signals. Applied Sciences. 2019;**9**:2870. DOI: 10.3390/app9142870

[107] Fernández A, López-Ibor M-I, Turrero A, et al. Lempel–Ziv complexity in schizophrenia: A MEG study. Clinical Neurophysiology. 2011;**122**:2227-2235. DOI: 10.1016/j.clinph.2011.04.011

[108] Dadgostar M, Setarehdan SK, Shahzadi S, Akin A. Classification of schizophrenia using SVM via FNIRS Biomedical Engineering: Applications. Basis and Communications. 2018;**30**:1850008. DOI: 10.4015/S1016237218500084

[109] Song H, Chen L, Gao R, et al. Automatic schizophrenic discrimination on fnirs by using complex brain network analysis and svm. BMC Medical Informatics and Decision Making. 2017;**17**:1-9. DOI: 10.1186/s12911-017-0559-5

[110] Yang H, Liu J, Sui J, Pearlson G, Calhoun VD. A hybrid machine learning method for fusing fmri and genetic data: Combining both improves classification of schizophrenia. Frontiers in Human Neuroscience. 2010;**4**:192. DOI: 10.3389/fnhum.2010.00192

[111] Rubia K, Russell T, Bullmore ET, et al. An FMRI study of reduced left prefrontal activation in schizophrenia during normal inhibitory function. Schizophrenia Research. 2001;**52**:47-55. DOI: 10.1016/S0920-9964(00)00173-0

[112] Veronese E, Castellani U, Peruzzo D, Bellani M, Brambilla P. Machine learning approaches: From theory to application in schizophrenia. Computational and Mathematical Methods in Medicine. 2013;**5**:1-12. DOI: 10.1155/2013/867924

[113] Starke G, De Clercq E, Borgwardt S, Elger BS. Computing schizophre-nia: Ethical challenges for machine learning in psychiatry. Psychological Medicine. 2020:1-7. DOI: 10.1017/S0033291720001683

[114] Cho GJ, Yim Y, Choi J, Ko SHL. Review of machine learning algorithms for diagnosing mental illness. Psychiatry Investigation. 2019;**16**:262. DOI: 10.30773/pi.2018.12.21.2

[115] Górriz JM, Ramírez J, Ortíz A, Martínez-Murcia FJ, Segovia F,

Suckling J, et al. Artificial intelligence within the interplay between natural and artificial computation. Advances in data science, trends and applications. Neurocomputing. 2020;**410**:237-270. DOI: 10.1016/j.neucom.2020.05.078

[116] Vieira S, Pinaya WH, Mechelli A. Using deep learning to investigate the neuroimaging correlates of psychiatric and neurological disorders: Methods and applications. Neuroscience and Biobehavioral Reviews. 2017;**2017**(74):58-75. DOI: 10.1016/j.neubiorev.2017.01.002

[117] Riaz A, Asad M, Alonso E, Slabaugh G. Deep fMRI: An end-to-end deep network for classification of fMRI data. In: Proc. 2018 IEEE 15th Int. Sym. on Biomedical Imaging, Washington, DC, USA. 2018. pp. 1419-1422

[118] Zou L, Zheng J, Miao C, Mckeown MJ, Wang ZJ. 3D CNN based automatic diagnosis of attention deficit hyperactivity disorder using functional and structural MRI. IEEE Access. 2017;**5**:23626-23636. DOI: 10.1109/ACCESS.2017.2762703

[119] Geng X, Xu J. Application of Autoencoder in Depression Diagnosis," in 2017 3rd Int. Conf. on Computer Science and Mechanical Automation, Wuhan, China, 2017

[120] Gadhoumi K, Lina JM, Mormann F, Gotman J. Seizure prediction for therapeutic devices: A review. Journal of Neuroscience Methods. 2016;**260**:270-282. DOI: 10.1016/j.jneumeth.2015.06.010

[121] Ambrosen KS, Skjerbæk MW, Foldager J, et al. A machine-learning framework for robust and reliable prediction of short- and long-term treatment response in initially antipsychotic-naïve schizophrenia patients based on multimodal neuropsychiatric data. Translational Psychiatry. 2020;**10**(276):2020. DOI: 10.1038/s41398-020-00962-8

[122] Alotaiby TN, Alshebeili SA, Alshawi T, Ahmad I, El-Samie FEA. EEG seizure detection and prediction algorithms: A survey. EURASIP Journal on Advances in Signal Processing. 2014;**183**. DOI: 10.1186/1687-6180-2014-183

[123] Zhou M, Tian C, Cao R, et al. Epileptic seizure detection based on EEG signals and CNN. Frontiers in Neuroinformatics. 2018;**12**:95. DOI: 10.3389/fninf.2018.00095

[124] Chen H, Song Y, Li X. Use of deep learning to detect personalized spatial-frequency abnormalities in EEGs of children with ADHD. Journal of Neural Engineering. 2019;**19**:066046. DOI: 10.1088/1741-2552/ab3a0a

[125] Ieracitano C, Mammone N, Bramanti A, Hussain A, Morabito FCA. A convolutional neural network approach for classification of dementia stages based on 2D-spectral representation of EEG recordings. Neurocomputing. 2019;**323**:96-107. DOI: 10.1016/j.neucom.2018.09.071

[126] Tibdewal MN, Dey HR, Mahadevappa M, Ray A, Malokar M. Multiple entropies performance measure for detection and localization of multi-channel epileptic EEG. Biomedical Signal Processing and Control. 2017;**38**:158-167. DOI: 10.1016/j.bspc.2017.05.002

[127] Xiang J, Tian C, Niu Y, Yan T, Li D, Cao R, et al. Abnormal entropy modulation of the eeg signal in patients with schizophrenia during the auditory paired-stimulus paradigm. Frontiers in Neuroinformatics. 2019;**19**:4. DOI: 10.3389/fninf.2019.00004

[128] Namazi H, Aghasian E, Ala TS. Fractal-based classification of electroencephalography (EEG) signals in healthy adolescents and adolescents with symptoms of schizophrenia. Technology and Health Care. 2019;**27**:233-241. DOI: 10.3233/THC-181497

[129] Takahashi T, Cho RY, Mizuno T, Kikuchi M, Murata T, Takahashi K, et al. Antipsychotics reverse abnormal EEG complexity in drug-naive schizophrenia: A multiscale entropy analysis. NeuroImage. 2010;**51**:173-182. DOI: 10.1016/j.neuroimage.2010.02.009

[130] LeCun Y, Bengio Y, Hinton G. Deep learning. Nature. 2015;**521**:436-444. DOI: 10.1038/nature14539

[131] Baevski A, Zhou Y, Mohamed A, Auli M. wav2vec 2.0: A Framework for Selfsupervised Learning of Speech Representations. Advances in neural information processing systems 33. In: 34th Conference on Neural Information Processing Systems (NeurIPS). Vancouver, Canada; 2020

[132] Arivazhagan N, Bapna A, Firat O, et al. Massively multilingual neural machine translation in the wild: Findings and challenges. arXiv preprint arXiv:1907.05019. 2019

[133] Brown TB, Mann B, Ryder N, et al. Language models are few-shot learners. arXiv preprint arXiv:2005.14165. 2020a

[134] Liu L, Ouyang W, Wang X, Fieguth P, Chen J, Liu X. Deep learning for generic object detection: A survey. International Journal of Computer Vision. 2020;**128**:261-318. DOI: 10.1007/s11263-019-01247-4

[135] Hornik K, Stinchcombe M, White H. Multilayer feedforward networks are universal approximators. Neural Networks. 1989;**2**:359-366. DOI: 10.1016/0893-6080(89)90020-8

[136] Schäfer AM, Zimmermann HG. Recurrent neural networks are universal approximators. International Journal of Neural Systems. 2007;**17**:253-263. DOI: 10.1142/S0129065707001111

[137] Elsken T, Metzen JH, Hutter F. Neural architecture search: A survey. arXiv preprint arXiv:1808.05377. 2018

[138] Zela A, Klein A, Falkner S, Hutter F. Towards automated deep learning: efficient joint neural architecture and hyperparameter search. arXiv preprint arXiv: 1807.06906. 2018

[139] Richards BA, Lillicrap TP, Beaudoin P, et al. A deep learning framework for neuroscience. Nature Neuroscience. 2019;**22**:1761-1770. DOI: 10.1038/s41593-019-0520-2

[140] Jose A, Nicolas I, Deepak C, Pablo E. Going deep into schizophrenia with artificial intelligence. Schizophrenia Research. 2022;**245**:122-140. DOI: 10.1016/j.schres.2021.05.018

[141] Broby D. Mark Zuckerberg wants to turn Facebook into a 'metaverse company' – what does that mean? The Conversation. Mark Zuckerberg wants to turn Facebook into a 'metaverse company' – what does that mean? 2021. available from: https://theconversation.com/mark-zuckerberg-wants-to-turn-facebook-into-a-metaverse-company-what-does-that-mean-165404#:~:text=In%20his%20quest%20to%20turn,avatars%20of%20themselves%20where%20appropriate. [Accessed: 2022.05.01]

[142] Peck T. Nick Clegg's outrageous defence of Facebook is enough to drive anyone to extreme. The Independent. Nick Clegg's outrageous defence of Facebook is enough to drive anyone to extremes The Independent. 2021. available from:

https://www.independent.co.uk/voices/nick-clegg-facebook-haugan-whistleblower-b1945055.html. [Accessed: 2022.05.01]

[143] Truzoli R, Osborne LA, Romano M, Reed P. The relationship between schizotypal personality and internet addiction in university students. Computers in Human Behavior. 2016;**63**:19-24. DOI: 10.1016/j.chb.2016.05.010

[144] Mittal VA, Tessner KD, Walker EF. Elevated social Internet use and schizotypal personality disorder in adolescents. Schizophrenia Research. 2007;**94**:50-57. DOI: 10.1016/j.schres.2007.04.009

[145] Tulay E, Metin B, Tarhan N, et al. Multimodal neuroimaging: Basic concepts and classification of neuropsychiatric diseases. Clinical EEG and Neuroscience. 2019;**50**:20-33. DOI: 10.1177/1550059418782093

[146] Rashid B, Calhoun V. Towards a brain-based predictor of mental illness. Human Brain Mapping. 2020;**41**:3468-3535

[147] Schlosser R, Nenadic J, Wagner G, et al. White matter abnormalities and brain activation in schizophrenia: A combined DTI and fMRI study. Schizophrenia Research. 2007;**89**:1-11

[148] Camchong J, MacDonald A, Bell C, et al. Altered functional and anatomical connectivity in schizophrenia. Schizophrenia Bulletin. 2011;**37**:640-650

[149] Koch K, Wagner G, Schachtzabel C, et al. Neural activation and radial diffusivity in schizophrenia: Combined fMRI and diffusion tensor imaging. 2011;**198**:223-229. DOI: 10.1192/bjp.bp.110.081836

[150] Isobe M, Miyata J, Hazama M, et al. Multimodal neuroimaging as a window into the pathological physiology of schizophrenia: Current trends and issues. Neuroscience Research. 2016;**102**:29-38. DOI: 10.1016/j.neures.2015.07.009

[151] Cetin M, Miyata J, Hazama M, et al. Multimodal based classification of schizophrenia patients. Conf Proc IEEE Eng Med Biology and Society. 2015;**2015**:2629-2632

Section 2

Diagnosis

Chapter 2

New Directions for Symptoms and Diagnosis in Schizophrenia

Bianca Daniela Crecan-Suciu and Ramona Păunescu

Abstract

Schizophrenia represents one challenging mental disorder from all the psychotic spectrum, considered to be a major health problem worldwide and because of the characteristic symptoms, the diagnosis is associated with high levels of stigmatization. It is quite common that the first acute symptoms to occur in early adult life and cause severe distress not only to the patient in need but also to their families. The schizophrenia clinical picture is usually misunderstood by the general public and consists of positive symptoms, negative symptoms, disorganized speech or behavior during a specific amount of time. In order to establish an accurate diagnosis, it requires taking into consideration both international classification systems, Diagnostic and Statistical Manual of Mental Disorders (DSM-5) and The International Classification of diseases (ICD-10), adding a fresh perspective to the newest chapter of ICD-11 called "Schizophrenia or other primary psychotic disorders", alongside with the diagnosis criteria, other new symptoms such as cognitive impairment emerge as an important feature of schizophrenia.

Keywords: Schizophrenia, positive symptoms, negative symptoms, classification systems, diagnosis

1. Introduction

A broad consensus points out that schizophrenia must be considered a complex mental disorder with an ongoing and rechanging hypothesis implying the possibility that diagnostic criteria could evolve during the course of new discoveries [1]. As we all know, most of the criteria characterizing schizophrenia are symptom-based, that usually rely on the psychiatrist's interpretation of what a patient defines as subjective experience, with no objective measures for a diagnostic test or even a biological marker, both of them could bring support in the clinical and treatment decision [2].

2. Defining schizophrenia from origins to the present

Regarding the terms melancholia or mania, the schizophrenia concept could be considered relatively recent from the mid-nineteenth century with the Morel cases as demence precoce and soon after appeared the Kraepelin integration under the name of dementia praecox, a term that included several clinical forms such as dementia praecox simplex, depressive dementia praecox, circular dementia praecox, agitated dementia praecox, periodic dementia praecox, but he was reserved regarding pathognomonic symptoms in schizophrenia [3]. Analyzing the symptoms, Bleuler suggested that the distinction between mandatory basic symptoms and accessory symptoms such as delusion and hallucinations are considered in the present time more important for the nosological systems as positive symptoms. On the other hand, Bleuler's perspective supposed that the basic symptoms were the most important such as thought and speech derailment, volitional ambivalence, affective incongruence, and withdrawal from what means reality [4]. Passing time, Kurt Schneider developed a prototype diagnostic criterion for schizophrenia, called the first-rank symptoms that included audible thoughts, voices arguing, discussing, commenting about the patient, experiences of influence on the body, interference or thought withdrawal, thought broadcast, and delusional perception. All these symptoms had high specificity and were later included in the ICD-10 classification [5].

3. New trends, innovations and changes in the diagnosis of schizophrenia

The need for a common language for reporting disorders all around the world concluded in development of two classifications systems called The International Classification of Diseases (ICD) and The Diagnosis and Statistical Manual of Mental Disorders (DSM), which one has several interrelated versions and the second one includes just a single set of operational diagnostic criteria to be used [6]. The presence of two different criteria sets for the same diagnoses emphasizes that definitions and concepts for psychiatric disorders are somewhat provisional and arbitrary in continuous development. During several editions, major differences were identified between this two, as ICD 10th version acknowledges schizophrenia as a group of disorders while DSM-IV describes a more unitary view of the illness [7]. Despite the evolution or the differences between the classification systems establishing a diagnosis of schizophrenia it still remains to present day a restricted overview of a clinical picture, describing different courses and outcomes based on characteristic symptoms that need to be present in a cross-section of the clinical picture, that vary differentially in weight of the diagnostic significance, mentioned as at least one or two or more, the duration of symptoms is also important, and the longitudinal course pattern [8]. As mentioned earlier, ICD-10 included the Schneider first rank symptoms as attributed high importance to this fact, but considered enough four weeks to eliminate acute, assumed non-schizophrenic episodes that could be induced by substance abuse [9]. The DSM-IV requires a more confident duration of at least six months that includes the prodromal and residual symptoms, implying that DSM has a tendency of selecting more severe cases in comparison with the ICD. Also, DSM in the B criteria mentions the need for a significant social and occupational dysfunction as an important definition criterion, but different view in the ICD as being context-dependent the level of dysfunctionality [10]. There is hope that making a diagnosis of schizophrenia should permit identifying the syndrome with adequate differentiation between degrees of symptom expression in patients and quantify the severity of the associated impairments. Regarding the evolution classification systems, it is mentioned two extremes courses in which there is complete recovery or worse evolution to continuous, unremitting symptoms that lead to serious deterioration. On the other hand, a major percent of schizophrenic patients manifest an episodic course with relapses and remissions, but it is worth mentioning a small percentage of those that recover very well [11]. The course pattern is not influenced by the symptoms, more important are the clinical onset, the duration of untreated psychosis, the comorbidity of substance abuse, and many else, but the characteristic symptoms tend to have predictive validity because just a small percentage of patients would be eventually reclassified into other mental illness categories cause as a clinical picture change [12].

Another perspective that needs to be mentioned is that of the choice between a categorical and a dimensional approach for the diagnosis of schizophrenia. The dimensional arrangement seems to have some difficulties, including an agreement on the number or nature of the dimension that needs to be established in order to be adequate for a clinically relevant variation, also there is not an empirically established grounded metric for the evaluation of severity or changes in psychotic disorders, and more important seems to be the complexity of dimensional concepts with different models in everyday clinical practice [13]. On the other hand, the categorical diagnosis represents an important tool for the clinicians, with precious information on the future relapse, recovery, risk of deterioration, and social disability, that play a role in the treatment decision with valuable data about similar patients in various communities. In this manner, the DSM-IV criteria for schizophrenia offers usefulness for predicting the outcome, because it implies some degree of chronicity, but considering schizophrenia on a spectrum may become more helpful in characterizing a syndrome with high heritability [14].

As the new approval of the 11th Revision of the ICD appeared, it raises new questions regarding the status of nosology of mental illnesses, and what changes have been made to the diagnostic guidelines. The principles underlying the revision of ICD-11 include global applicability that refers to the cultural diversity of the new version of ICD-11 must incorporate, also scientific validity as it is established as a State-of-the-Art in terms of research and classification of mental pathologies and clinical utility by including the accuracy of descriptions, the ease of application, the time required for use and the need to select appropriate therapeutic and management decisions [15]. The ICD-11 includes a flexible, alphanumeric coding named BLOCK, and its use allows a larger diagnostic grouping, based on scientific evidence and clinical needs. The ICD-11 includes 28 chapters, with 6 chapters in addition to the old version of ICD-10. In the previous version of ICD-11, the number of groups was restricted by a decimal coding system, thus allowing a maximum of 10 pathological groups included, resulting in the loss of scientific relevance and clinical utility [16]. The organization of the ICD-10 reflects the original conceptualization of the Kraepelin Textbook of Psychiatry, but ICD-11 tries to order the diagnostic groups in chapter 06 called Mental, behavioral or neurodevelopmental disorders from a developmental perspective and brings them together diagnoses according to etiological, psychopathological, and phenomenological characteristics. Regarding the composition of the ICD-11 structure, the American Psychiatric Association also had a great influence, wanting to increase the concordance between ICD-11 and DSM-5 [17]. It is important to mention the main objectives for the DSM-5 diagnostic guide for Mental Disorders such as clinical utility, with its considerations being the facilitation of evaluation in the clinical routine, providing clarity in distinguishing the various psychiatric disorders, and only additionally, it provides research support for a better understanding of the cause and psycho-pathogenic pathways, also the organization reflects the process of development and evolution throughout life. Multiple comparative studies have reported positive evaluations by clinicians in terms of clinical utility, reliability, and diagnostic process quality for the ICD-11 system compared to ICD-10

[18]. In ICD-11 it has replaced the chapter from ICD 10—Schizophrenia, schizotypal disorders, and delusional disorders with—Schizophrenia or other primary psychotic disorders (BlockL1-6A2) and is the second chapter in the list of nosological classes, following chapter Neurodevelopmental disorders. Different from ICD-10 where it was preceded by Organic Mental Disorders and Substance Use Disorders. In ICD-11 the term Spectrum is not used, as in DSM-5 (Schizophrenia Spectrum Disorders and Other Psychotic Disorders) for class labeling. Research places many disturbances across a spectrum, namely very close illnesses that have in common symptoms, risk factors, neural substrate, and this spectrum concept actually accepts that the boundaries between the disturbances are much more flexible and vaguely defined [19].

Starting from the hypothesis that the diagnosis of Schizophrenia and the initiation of treatment is made relatively late, thus explaining the unfavorable evolution. It is proposed to introduce the diagnosis of Attenuated Psychosis in the DSM-5, thus providing the framework and support for clinicians in recognizing and monitoring psychotic symptoms from the earliest stages of manifestation with a desire to obtain a practice of rapid and early intervention [20]. It was proposed to introduce this construct in ICD-11, but it was abandoned, the reason was the increased prevalence in establishing the diagnosis of psychosis because there is a percentage of vulnerable individuals at risk but who will not develop criteria for a clear diagnosis of schizophrenia, attracting a high degree of stigma [21].

The term "primary" in the name chapter from the ICD-11 classification system, indicates that psychotic processes are the core feature of these disorders, in contrast to other mental disorders that may be associated with psychotic symptoms, but they occur as a result of other psychopathological mechanisms involved. It can be assumed that this term refers to the clinical construct that has no correspondence at the level of biological or genetic markers, and the actual cause remains still unknown even today [22].

Defining schizophrenia from origins to the present time includes mentioning that the construct of Schizophrenia in ICD-10 and DSM-IV-TR derives from the Kraepelin formulation of praecox dementia, with two distinct patterns of evolution, first one as Dementia praecox, the other one as Manic-depressive psychosis. Also, Bleuler considers a group of schizophrenia, having in common the split of mental functions (fundamental and accessory symptoms), in association with Schneider's first-order symptoms [23]. As we can conclude the current definition of Schizophrenia in ICD and DSM includes the chronicity of Kraepelin, the Bleuler negative symptoms, and Schneider's positive symptoms. But in ICD-11, the importance given to Schneider symptoms of the first rank is abandoned, although they remain unchanged, they are considered of the same importance as the rest of the positive symptoms. The consideration of this change stands because they are not being considered specific and pathognomonic, and the delimitation between bizarre and non-bizarre is difficult to estimate [24]. The impact of this change will be reduced, as a reflection of the prevalence of diagnosis, because most studies estimate that less than 5% of those diagnosed with Schizophrenia would have obtained it only in the presence of a single bizarre delusional idea [25]. Moreover, the distinction between delirium and phenomena of control or xenopathic influence on the self is kept, as considered core symptoms. An innovation brought by ICD-11 is the introduction in the description of the disorder of cognitive deficits, as characteristic symptoms of Schizophrenia, but with no clarifications to be provided regarding the issue of prodromal, active, or residual phases [26].

ICD-10 views Schizophrenia as a group of disorders, while DSM-IV describes it as a unitary condition, but in ICD-11-Schizophrenia is presented simpler, as the clinical forms from the ICD-10 are abandoned, an aspect also found in DSM-5 due to the lack of clinical subtypes. The elimination of these subtypes was decided due to the belief that they offer a weak heterogeneity of the disorder, with low longitudinal stability, as the research does not confirm their predictive validity, and also, they do not exert influences on the therapeutic approach [27]. Studies show in their current clinical practice a reduced use of them, only the paranoid and undifferentiated subtype registered a more frequent use, as paranoid ideas are considered nonspecific, and can be found in affective episodes, delusional disorders, or dementia [28].

The past construct was considered inadequate to describe the evolutionary stages and psychopathological dimension of schizophrenia. For this reason, a set of dimensional ratings has been introduced, for a better description of the symptomatic manifestations, they can be applied only after the formulation of the diagnoses. It is considered of little importance to focus on the diagnostic categories when the dimensional classification is the one that focuses on the relevant aspects of the current clinical presentation, as well as the recovery [29]. Dimensional specifications of the evolution were also introduced, in order to emphasize the existence of different clinical-evolutionary profiles of a unique disorder. This draws attention to distinct profiles of the manifestation of the same disorder. Importance is given to the differentiation between the first episode of Schizophrenia, and subsequent, multiple episodes, in partial or complete remission, or on a continuous evolution, thus implying the need to establish a diagnosis as early as possible [30].

4. Old and new symptoms in Schizophrenia

Along with the diagnosis criteria, both DSM-5 and ICD-11 have introduced a symptom specifier which replaced the subtypes of schizophrenia in the case of ICD. The specifier records information on the presence or absence of symptoms, their longitudinal course, response to treatment, and prognosis for the disorder [31]. The specifier must be constantly assessed throughout the course of the disease, and it determines the severity of clinical manifestations between patients and in the same patient at different episodes. For ICD-11 the specifier categories include positive, negative, depressive, manic, psychomotor, and cognitive deficits while DSM-5 splits positive symptoms and consider individually hallucinations, delusions, and disorganized course.

Positive symptoms were always the most evident features of schizophrenia and contributed highly to the stigma associated with illness. Positive symptoms include a wide palette of delusions, hallucinations that can involve one or several sensory receptors, disorganized thinking, passivity experiences, and altered behavior.

4.1 Delusions

Delusions are defined as false ideas or beliefs that cannot be attributed to the patient's educational, social, or cultural background, that are not amenable to logic, and of which the patient is strongly convinced. Delusions have been divided into primary and secondary delusions. Primary delusions, which are more characteristic of schizophrenia, do not occur in response to other psychiatric symptoms such as hallucinations. Secondary delusions are subsequent to other psychopathology (e.g. hallucinations or mood disorder) and are thus understandable in circumstances of the person's background culture, or emotional state [32]. Delusions in schizophrenia vary in content (e.g. persecutory, grandiose, religious, self-referential) and may present as monothematic or polythematic; they can be correlated with hallucinations and can severely impact other mental aspects of the individual (e.g. mood, behavior). Other characteristics such as levels of conviction, preoccupation (subjugation of behavior), and distress should be considered when examining delusions. These features are also key aspects that can help distinguish between an over-valued belief and a delusional one. Studies show that 70% of patients experience persecutory delusions and 67% experience self-referential delusions [33]. Delusions have different degrees of organization. Some delusions are simple, whereas others are very complex and involve many people or organizations. Some delusions have a stable time course and may last for many years, while others are present for a short time. Studies suggest that certain factors such as single life, older age, delusions of being controlled, delusional behavior, and higher levels of psychopathology and functional impairment are associated with the persistence of delusional thinking [34].

4.2 Hallucinations

Hallucinations are defined as percepts, experienced by a person, in the absence of an appropriate stimulus from the outside world. In patients with schizophrenia auditory hallucinations are by far the most common, followed by visual hallucinations, and then by tactile and olfactory or gustatory hallucinations [35]. Hallucinations can involve one or more receptors and can occur unilaterally or bilaterally. They may be simple or complex and may have a laudatory, hostile, or imperative character. Studies suggest that the prevalence of hallucinations in multiple sensory modalities seems to be the most frequent perceptual symptom of patients diagnosed with a schizophrenia spectrum disorder. The same data showed that hallucinations experienced in a single sensory modality (especially auditory ones) increase the risk for the occurrence of more sensory perception disturbances [36].

Auditory hallucinations (AHs) are defined as experiences without an external stimulus with individuals perceiving voices distinct from their own thoughts, whether the voices are familiar or not. They are considered a main positive symptom of schizophrenia [37]. AHs are found with a lifetime prevalence rate of 60–80% in schizophrenia spectrum disorders [38] and a 1-year prevalence rate of 50–70% in schizophrenia specifically [39]. AHs may have a severe negative impact on one's mental health, for instance, increasing depressive symptoms and leading to suicidal ideation or attempt [36, 40].

Visual hallucinations are the second most common type of perception disturbances in schizophrenia with an estimated mean prevalence of 27% [39]. Visual hallucinations are not the only form of perceptual anomaly encountered in schizophrenia. Studies pointed out that over 60% of schizophrenic patients experience visual distortions involving changes in clarity, form, brightness, color, motion, or persistence of visual stimuli [41–44]. It has also been reported that visual imagery is increased in people with schizophrenia [45]. The presence of VH in psychosis has often been linked to a more severe psychopathological profile. In schizophrenia VHs typically co-occur in association with other hallucinations and other sensory modalities [46]. Studies reported that co-occurring visual and auditory hallucinations occur in up to 84% of individuals with schizophrenia [39].

Tactile and somatic hallucinations are the third most common type of perceptual disturbances presented in schizophrenia with a prevalence ranging from 4 to 25% across studies [46]. Tactile and somatic hallucinations are classified as bodily hallucinations, a term that also includes a wide group of corporeal sensations such as sexual hallucinations, coenesthesiopathies, proprioceptive hallucinations, kinesthetic hallucinations, vestibular hallucinations, hallucinated pain, and thermal hallucinations [47]. Tactile hallucinations are also called haptic hallucinations and are defined as sensations of touch in the absence of a stimulus from the outside world. They can present as an apparent touch to the skin, a sting, a hand on one's shoulder, or a blow to the face. From a pathophysiological perspective, they are associated with activity in sensory cortical areas subserving the skin and subcutaneous tissues. Somatic hallucinations are defined as bodily sensations experienced inside the body, in the absence of an objectifiable source or cause [48]. Although the data on this type of hallucination is scarce, studies have suggested a correlation between tactile hallucinations and longer duration and severity of the illness [46, 49]. Sexual hallucinations, as a subtype of tactile and somatic hallucinations, are probably the most neglected types of hallucination. This may be due to several reasons involving the clinician who might not ask for information on perceptual disturbances that fall outside the five basic sensory modalities (i.e. olfaction, taste, vision, audition, and touch) and the patients suffering from sexual hallucinations who might be ashamed to talk about these phenomena [47].

Olfactory (OHs) and gustatory hallucinations are frequently associated, and they represent other types of hallucinations in schizophrenic patients. The prevalence of olfactory hallucinations ranges from 15% to 27%, while for gustatory hallucinations the prevalence is estimated from 4% to 14% [48]. Both types of hallucinations can occur as negative or positive ones. The most common negative olfactory hallucinations include odors of blood, smoke, burnt rubber, or feces while positive odors are fruity and perfume-like [50]. Sociocultural factors may modulate the self-reporting and/or detection of OHs and hallucinations in other modalities. Referential/control delusions promote the generation and/or maintenance of OHs independent of factors shared with other hallucinations. OHs and hallucinations of taste, touch, and bodily sensation frequently co-occur [51]. Studies focusing on OHs found no relationship between disease severity measures and type or frequency of OHs but reported significant relationships between frequency of OHs and severity of tactile hallucinations. Although the predominance of negative OHs was noted, there were also many reports of positive OHs [50].

Multimodal hallucinations may be defined as anomalous perceptions occurring in two or more sensory systems, concurrently or serially in time, not necessarily sharing a single source, origin, or thematic content [52]. Recent evidence suggests that multimodal hallucinations are more common than previously recognized and have a greater negative impact than unimodal hallucinations. For example, recent evidence shows that 36–81% of patients with schizophrenia spectrum disorders experience multimodal hallucination [53]. When compared to unimodal experiences, multimodal hallucinations in clinical samples have been associated with increased levels of distress, negative affect, illness severity, and traumatic events [54, 55]. Research showed that patients with late-onset schizophrenia are considered to complain more of visual, tactile, and olfactory hallucinations, third-person running commentary, and accusatory or abusive auditory hallucinations, than early-onset patients [56]. Regarding accompanying symptoms, all types of hallucinations seem to be associated with other clinical features. Thus, the study of Melvin et al. [57] reported clusters of emotional feelings associated with hallucinations which by order of frequency could be described as fear and anxiety; despair and powerlessness; abused and threat; frustration and anger; loneliness; stress and distress and worry. The same research highlighted co-occurring bodily feelings such as tension, pressure, agitation, chills, heaviness, and dizziness, across hallucination types identifiable, localized, specific, and communicable. The most involved body areas included the head and shoulders followed by the chest, abdomen, and legs and these corporeal sensations arose across hallucination types.

Few studies focused on the trajectories of hallucinations over the years. Ten years follow-up of auditory hallucinations in schizophrenia yield several important clinical implications. The results of the study suggested that the majority of patients with schizophrenia improve on auditory hallucinations during the first ten years with most patients improving within the first year. Another finding established a relationship between the presence of an alcohol abuse disorder and a longer DUP at treatment initiation and a worse course of auditory hallucinations over time [58]. Another study that included a 20 year follow-up period reported a decrease in both auditory and visual hallucinations over time with auditory hallucinations being more common than visual hallucinations, especially during the early years and throughout the course of the illness [59]. Within the study population, olfactory hallucination occurred at a low rate in schizophrenia patients during the 20-year follow-up, ranging from 0 to 11%. In terms of recovery prediction, auditory hallucinations were associated with being less likely to have a recovery over the next 20 years. The same authors pointed out that 44% of schizophrenia patients showed frequent or chronic hallucinations over the 20-year course of the study. The early presence of hallucinations predicted the lack of a future period of recovery in all patients, and increased hallucinatory activity was associated with reduced work attainment in all patients [60].

4.3 Disorganization

Another important factor that has received increasing attention in schizophrenia is disorganization with both disorganized thinking and behavior representing diagnosis criteria. The disorganization dimension was firstly introduced by Liddle [61] who identified inappropriate effect, poverty of content of speech, and formal thought disorder as component items using clinical assessment scales. Over time, research confirmed disorganization as a separate symptom dimension with respect to the positive one, with distinct associations with the course and outcome of schizophrenia [62, 63]. The Positive and Negative Syndrome Scale [PANSS] factorial analyses have identified different items, such as "conceptual disorganization", "difficulty in abstract thinking", "poor attention", "disorientation", "mannerism and posturing" and "stereotyped thinking", as component items of the disorganization dimension [64, 65]. Disorganization symptoms are found to be inversely associated with long-term functioning. Several studies showed a strong inverse correlation between disorganization and social functions emphasizing that the more symptomatic the patients are, the greater the difficulties in real-world functioning and performance [66, 67]. A large study investigating the role of illness-related factors on the global functioning in patients with schizophrenia observed a key role in the illness-related variables' disorganization. Defining the structure of the Positive and Negative Syndrome Scale (PANSS) disorganization dimension according to the consensus 5-factor solution proposed by Wallwork et al. [68] the results of the analysis pointed to an overlap that cannot be underestimated for the items "difficulties in abstract thinking" and "poor attention" with neurocognitive impairment. The authors also underlined those positive symptoms and disorganization proved to have significant direct and indirect effects on real-life functioning [69]. Ventura et al. [70] hypothesized that the close link between disorganization and functional outcomes may be due to the impact of disorganization symptoms on communication and social interactions, as well as to the lack of compensatory mechanisms. Moreover, it has been suggested that symptoms such as incoherent thinking and speech can "mask" delusions and hallucinations. Other disorganization symptoms such as conceptual disorganization, loose associations, disrupted goal-directed sequencing, and circumstantiality, were found to have direct implications for community activities [69]. Disorganization dimension is also in relationship with neurocognitive functioning and studies observed that disorganization had a stronger impact on neurocognition than positive or negative symptoms [71–73]. In their meta-analysis, Ventura et al. [70] reported that disorganization was related to all domains of neurocognitive functioning including speed of processing, attention/vigilance, working memory, verbal learning, visual learning, reasoning, and problem-solving and social cognition). Specific items on PANSS such as "Conceptual disorganization" (P2) were reported as the item that correlated more than others with neurocognitive dysfunction. For the component item "Difficulty in abstract thinking" (N5) only a moderate association with the neurocognitive composite score was found [74]. Findings showed that patients experiencing first episode of schizophrenia (FES) have relevant levels of disorganized symptoms. Disorganization seems to show greater psychopathological affinities with negative symptoms than with positive symptoms with a putative potentiating detrimental effect on daily functioning and social interaction. Authors pointed out that evidence of significant baseline correlations between disorganization and other PANSS domains suggests that it may be an early clinical feature of general severity in FES psychopathology [75]. Disorganization criteria seem to play a role key also in the cases of treatment resistant schizophrenia. A recent study identified a higher severity of conceptual disorganization difficulty in abstract thinking and unusual thought content items within PANSS to be predictive of treatment resistance to schizophrenia [76]. Although the disorganized dimension is the least studied when compared to the positive and negative dimensions of the PANSS, there is consistent evidence for the clinical impact of disorganization and its correlates in neurocognition, genetics, and neuroimaging [77].

Disorganized behavior and deficits in adaptive goal-directed behavior contribute to disability in schizophrenia [78]. Behavioral abnormalities may include context-inappropriate commission errors that may appear bizarre and out of place [79]. Similar to the explanation for the disorganized speech in schizophrenia, behavioral disorganization may be a manifestation of an underlying abnormality of the neural activity supporting a specific type of conceptual knowledge encoding goal-related requirements of behavioral actions. Execution and comprehension of behavior may share neural systems subserving real-world knowledge and particularly more complex, non-routine tasks, such planning may depend on a neural system [80–83]. Several psychopathology-based models tried to provide an integrative theoretical approach to the study of goal-directed behaviors. An initial bidimensional model proposed by Frith, [84] which is based on the distinction between positive and negative symptoms of schizophrenia, represents the most useful framework for the clinical, theoretical, and epistemological study of goal-directed actions. According to Frith, there are two main paths of action: those produced in response to environmental stimuli and those driven by a goal and a willed intention to act. The model proposes that impairments in these two paths may differ according to the dominant symptoms in people with schizophrenia. When negative symptoms are dominant, people with schizophrenia may have trouble connecting their goals and plans with the intention to act, thus leading to a failure of self-initiated actions. Instead, when positive symptoms are dominant, stimulus-driven actions are disinhibited, leading to abnormal or perseverative behaviors. The Hardy-Baylé model [85] suggests that disorganized symptoms may be specifically linked to impairments in contextual processing leading to impaired social behaviors. A common impairment in goal-directed behaviors in people with schizophrenia is a deficit in the perception and contextual integration of others' actions with a tendency to perceive specific events rather than units of interconnected behaviors relevant to the achievement of a goal, deficits that are associated with more severe disorganized symptoms [86, 87].

4.4 Passivity symptoms

Passivity experiences are hallmark symptoms of schizophrenia. They are characterized by the belief that one's thoughts or actions are influenced or controlled by an external agent. From this point of view, psychotic passivity experiences can be generally understood as a failure of the causal association between internal representations of action programs and the perception of external changes resulting from those actions [88]. Recent psychopathological models underlined the perceptual features of passivity experiences. These models suggest that passivity experiences in schizophrenia generally arise from dysfunctional processing of sensory perceptions resulting from own actions [89–91]. In accordance with this model, the action monitoring approach might provide a pathophysiological model of the self-monitoring failure involved not only in passivity experiences but also in other schizophrenic symptoms like, for example, auditory hallucinations which are possibly linked to defective monitoring of speech production [88, 92]. The feeling of control over own actions and their consequences, also known as the sense of agency, is thought to comprise multiple inter-related elements [93]. One element, self-agency, is the subjective awareness that one has initiated and executed one's actions, while other-agency is the representation of events caused by another person or agent [94]. Research pointed out that individuals with schizophrenia and passivity symptoms make many errors on motor tasks that measure agency when reporting the agent of their actions [88, 91]. These agency errors are thought to be caused by abnormal internal timing processes in schizophrenia [95]. Timing mechanisms are the neurological and neuropsychological processes that dictate the internal experience of the flow of time and play a key role in the coordination of neural circuits and events [96, 97]. Normal internal timing has an important role in the coordination of action elements and correct agency attributions [98]. Patients with schizophrenia and passivity symptoms have impaired timing and a broader perceptual binding window for sensory events when making action decisions, resulting in altered sensitivity to temporal incongruence. Along with internal timing problems that contribute to excessive associability with external sensory stimuli studies show that passivity symptoms are linked to deficits in body representations encompassing body image and body schema and changes in the sense of agency [99, 100].

4.5 Negative symptoms

Negative symptoms are defined as a weakening or absence of normal behaviors and functions related to motivation and interest, or verbal/emotional expression. The negative symptom domain consists of five key constructs: blunted affect, alogia (reduction in quantity of words spoken), avolition (reduced goal-directed activity due to decreased motivation), asociality, and anhedonia (reduced experience of pleasure). Negative symptoms are common in schizophrenia and can occur at any point in the course of illness, although they are reported as the most common first symptom of schizophrenia [101]. Their prevalence in first-episode psychosis is high, 50–90% and 20–40% of schizophrenia patients have persisting negative symptoms [102]. Studies show that the majority of the patients diagnosed with schizophrenia spectrum disorders have at least one negative symptom while 41% of the patients present at least two negative symptoms [103]. In a 15-year prospective study of patients with schizophrenia, schizoaffective and affective disorders, the prevalence of negative symptoms was found to be as high as 75% for the first diagnosis category [104]. Moreover, negative symptoms along with other nonspecific clinical symptoms, such as depression, anxiety symptoms, social isolation, and school/occupational failure are often present during the prodromal phase of schizophrenia [105]. In a retrospective study assessing the onset of schizophrenia, negative symptoms were observed in 95% of patients seeking psychiatric assistance. Furthermore, in the pre-symptomatic phase of the disease, 32.7% of the subjects demonstrated social withdrawal with increasing self-isolation, 25.8% developed asthenoneurotic and asthenodepressive symptoms, and only 7% showed apatho-abulic manifestation [106]. The term negative symptom is a general, descriptive term that does not involve considerations about the symptom cause, longitudinal stability, or duration. Contrarily, primary and secondary negative symptoms refer to distinct subgroups of negative symptoms differing in their cause, longitudinal stability, or duration and differentiated through longitudinal observation. Primary and enduring negative symptoms refer to the symptoms that are intrinsic to schizophrenia, while secondary negative symptoms refer to negative symptoms occurring in association with, or presumably caused by, positive symptoms, affective symptoms, medication side effects, environmental factors, or other treatment- and illness-related aspects. The term deficit symptoms are used to refer to those negative symptoms that are present as enduring symptoms, present during and between episodes of positive symptom exacerbation, and observable regardless of the patient's medication status; they are caused by a specific disease process that is separate from the genetic and neurobiological factors that contribute to nondeficit schizophrenia [107, 108]. The deficit syndrome appears to remain stable throughout the course of illness, occurring in approximately 15% of patients experiencing the first episode of schizophrenia and in 15–20% of all cases of schizophrenia [109, 110]. In contrast to all other variants of the disease, patients with deficit schizophrenia consistently demonstrate the worst therapeutic and social prognosis [111]. Several studies confirmed a two-factor structure of negative symptoms (motivational-volitional and emotional-expressive disorders) which seems to be supported by the trajectory of their development in the course of the disease, including their long-term stability and relationship with functional outcomes [112, 113]. This classification may be explained by possible different neurophysiological and neurochemical mechanisms [114]. The severity of negative symptoms in schizophrenia has been linked to worse functional outcomes in areas such as occupational and academic performance, household integration, social functioning, and quality of life [115]. Also, a relationship between specific negative symptoms and impaired functioning has been outlined. Thus, avolition has been proposed as a key negative symptom construct related to functional deterioration while loss of motivation is thought to be associated with changes in social behaviors [101, 115]. Although the distinction between primary and secondary negative symptoms is important, managing negative symptoms and differentiating between the two categories of symptoms in schizophrenia is a major challenge for psychiatric services [116].

4.6 Psychomotor disturbances

The most common psychomotor disturbances encountered in schizophrenia are catatonic restlessness or agitation, posturing, waxy flexibility, negativism, mutism, or stupor [117]. Catatonia is a clinical syndrome characterized by the presence of multiple psychomotor disturbances. Catatonic phenomena comprise more than 40 affective, behavioral, and motor symptoms (e.g. stupor, mutism, waxy flexibility, rigidity, posturing, mannerism, negativism, and stereotypy) [118, 119]. The syndrome may present in two different subtypes: hypokinetic or retarded catatonia and hyperkinetic or excited catatonia. The hypokinetic type is associated with signs reflecting a paucity of movement, including immobility, staring, mutism, rigidity, and reduced oral intake, along with more bizarre features such as posturing, grimacing, negativism, waxy flexibility, echolalia or echopraxia, stereotypy and verbigeration [120]. Excited catatonia, on the other hand, is characterized by severe psychomotor agitation potentially leading to life-threatening complications such as hyperthermia, altered consciousness, and autonomic dysfunction [121]. Research reported a prevalence of catatonia in schizophrenia of 9.8% [122]. The outbreak of catatonia is usually acute, in a matter of hours or days, resulting in frequent use of the emergency departments and hospitalisation. However, in schizophrenia, the syndrome may have a subacute onset and a tendency to become chronic [123].

Mutism is an inability or unwillingness to speak, resulting in an absent or marked lack of verbal output. Similar to other symptoms within psychomotor disturbances, mutism rarely occurs as a single feature. It is commonly seen in association with disturbances in behavior, thought processes, affect, or level of consciousness [124]. Data from literature suggest that mutism in schizophrenia can be a consequence of positive symptoms (i.e. secondary to other psychotic symptoms like delusions and hallucinations, e.g., due to hallucinations commanding the patient to not speak) or part of disorganized behavior (i.e. as an extreme form of alogia). Mutism might develop in a patient, even involuntarily, to mitigate the distress caused by paranoid delusions or hallucinations or to disguise the illness and reduce the associated stigma [125]. A recent report suggests that religion and the psychological uses of silence appear to play a part in the occurrence of the symptom of mutism [126].

4.7 Psychomotor slowing

Psychomotor slowing (hypokinesia) is defined as a reduction in the initiation, amount, or speed of movement, slowness in planning and execution of motor tasks, and as a decrease in the total quantity of activities. This slowing in actions co-occurs with other motor symptoms such as spontaneous involuntary movements (e.g. dyskinesias) and is a core feature of the disorder that is present across the different stages of schizophrenia (i.e. prodromal, first episode, chronic stage) [127–129]. Psychomotor planning present in the early stages of schizophrenia involves deficient planning in motor sequences but intact motor action [130]. Patients diagnosed with schizophrenia can be observed to have longer thinking latencies and to be slowed in their responses or in their movements. In more severely affected patients, movements can be extremely slow, and psychomotor activity is sometimes reduced to the bare minimum, affecting their social-communicative interactions and daily-life activities. Both gross and fine motor performances have been reported to be affected [131]. The current state of knowledge suggests that psychomotor slowing in schizophrenia is related to a disturbance in cortico-subcortical interaction within the motor loop compensated by premotor cortical activity [132]. Hypokinesia is frequently correlated with negative symptoms (avolition) and with parkinsonian signs [133]. Evidence suggests that psychomotor slowing is present in unaffected first-degree relatives and twins of patients and that it is associated with both symptoms and relevant structural and functional abnormalities across the schizophrenia spectrum, indicating that this feature may be a key endophenotype for schizophrenia. General psychomotor slowing in psychosis was found to become progressively worse from the prodromal stage to chronic schizophrenia [134]. Studies showed that hypokinesia is a prognostic factor for poor social, functional, and clinical outcomes [131].

4.8 Affective symptoms

In addition to positive, negative, and disorganization, patients with schizophrenia often exhibit affective symptoms, including depression and anxiety. Affective symptoms in schizophrenia can be particularly disturbing for the patients increasing the risk of suicide and diminishing quality of life [135]. Because of the frequent overlap between the negative symptoms and affective symptoms, it can be often difficult to distinguish between the two domains, especially when it comes to depressive symptoms. Studies pointed out that depressive symptoms may be present in as many as 80% of patients with schizophrenia while symptoms of mania are reported in as many as 20% of individuals with schizophrenia [136]. Despite this fact, only 10–30% of patients with schizophrenia spectrum disorders meet criteria for the schizoaffective disorder [137], with a significant proportion of patients meeting diagnostic criteria for both schizophrenia and mood disorders. A recent meta-analysis reported a prevalence of 28.6% for comorbid depression in schizophrenia [138]. In addition to patients who meet criteria for major depression, there are also a significant number of patients with schizophrenia who experience subsyndromal depressive symptoms. A study including a large, multicenter sample of older adults with schizophrenia spectrum disorder found that 78.1% of older adults had either subsyndromal or syndromal depressive symptoms with a higher prevalence of subsyndromal depressive in individuals with an onset of schizophrenia spectrum disorder before 40 years of age than in those with an age at onset between 40 and 60 years [139]. The most prevalent depressive symptoms reported in individuals with schizophrenia were depressed mood, morning depression, diminished work and activities, guilt, anergia, psychological anxiety, observed depression, initial insomnia, and hopelessness [140]. Up-to-date literature highlighted that comorbid depressive symptoms are present in all phases of schizophrenia [141] and they correlated with a higher risk of suicide [142, 143], worse psychosocial functioning [144], and poorer quality of life [145].

4.9 Cognitive symptoms

Although cognitive impairment is not among the diagnostic criteria in schizophrenia it is considered to be a core feature of schizophrenia. Deficits are moderate to severe across several domains, including attention, working memory, verbal learning and memory, executive functions, and social cognition. These deficits pre-date the onset of frank psychosis and are stable throughout the course of the illness in most patients [146]. The presence of cognitive deficits observed from the first episode of the illness suggests they are not due to exposure to neuroleptic medication [147]. Results from studies assessing the longitudinal changes in cognition for patients with schizophrenia support the presence of a cognitive decline that progresses after the psychosis onset.

Thus, a recent study with 10 years of prospective follow-up of patients with first-episode psychosis found a progressive decline in IQ and in specific neurocognitive domains, such as verbal knowledge and memory in patients who were later diagnosed with schizophrenia [148]. Neurocognitive impairment in schizophrenia is also shown to be associated with neroanatomical alterations. A recent study demonstrated that cortical thickness in bilateral superior frontal and right transverse temporal regions correlates positively with cognitive performance (particularly attention/vigilance) suggesting that thickness in these regions is of specific importance for cognitive performance in schizophrenia, possibly reflecting compensatory processes [149]. The prevalence of cognitive impairments in patients with schizophrenia is high, with more than 80% of patients showing significant impairment [150]. Mascio et al. [151] reported a prevalence of 55% for one or more cognitive problems and a prevalence of 60% for at least one cognitive domain impairment in their large sample study. The cognitive dysfunctions within the research were also strongly correlated with several socio-demographic factors (gender, education, ethnicity, marital status, and employment) as well as adverse clinical outcomes.

Attention deficits are reported among most pervasive neurocognitive features and have a role in predicting functional outcomes. The components most studied in schizophrenia are selective attention and sustained attention. Attention operates to activate processes that enhance the processing of relevant signals, inhibits irrelevant signals in a way that strengthens resistance to interference and distractibility, and coordinates the realization of concurrent tasks by distributing processing resources. Decreased inhibition of interfering information seems to be a hallmark of cognitive disturbances in schizophrenia [152].

Memory is the cognitive area showing the most pronounced deficits with working memory and episodic memory appearing to be the most impaired. Working memory has been defined as the ability to transiently hold and manipulate information to guide goal-directed behavior. Its contents are constitutively updated, monitored, and manipulated in response to immediate processing demands [153]. Results from a large meta-analysis pointed to working memory deficits in task performance for patients with schizophrenia in all modalities examined showing that these deficits are robust across different tasks, modalities, and subject variables, though there appear to be more consistent and greater impairments in the visuospatial domain than other domains [154]. Similarly, another meta-analysis found statistically significant impairment across the domains of phonological, visuospatial, and central executive working memory, deficits which were not explained by discrepancies in current IQ between schizophrenia and control groups, duration of illness, or use of antipsychotic medications [155]. The working memory impairments appear to reflect alterations in the neural circuitry of the dorsolateral (DLPFC) prefrontal cortex [156]. Findings from multiple studies have clearly implicated pathology of the dorsolateral prefrontal cortex (DLPFC) as playing a central role in the pathophysiology of SZ, particularly with regard to key cognitive features such as deficits in working memory and cognitive control [157]. Working memory deficits, particularly in terms of impaired encoding and maintenance, are found in a disproportionate number of schizophrenia patients. Studies indicate that impaired working memory is a trait characteristic of schizophrenia and present from the prodrome to the chronic stages of the disorder. There is also evidence that working memory impairment is genetically transmitted and also present in unaffected relatives of schizophrenia probands at a higher rate than in the general population. All those factors lead to the assumption that working memory impairment is an excellent candidate for endophenotypic marker status in terms of schizophrenia liability [158]. Episodic memory is a category of long-term memory defined as a record of a person's experience that includes temporally dated information and spatio-temporal relations [159]. Episodic memory is a cognitive area that is consistently impaired in schizophrenia from prodromal to chronic phases but is also found in first- and second-degree relatives of patients. Episodic memory impairment was linked to deficits in both encoding and retrieval processes [160]. Context processing in episodic memory reflects the ability to encode and retrieve relationships among event features, such as when, where, and with whom they occurred. Research suggested that disruptions in such processing may underlie the episodic memory impairments observed in schizophrenia [161, 162]. Magnetic resonance imaging studies revealed an apparent disruption in frontotemporal connectivity connected to episodic memory dysfunctions [163].

4.10 Executive functions

The term executive functions comprise a diverse set of cognitive capacities meant to guide, monitor, and control our actions and mental processes to meet particular goals in a purposeful manner. Executive functions may be defined as higher-order neurocognitive functions consisting of abilities to plan and structure goal-directed activity and problem-solving behavior in a strategic, flexible manner or as merely the ability to respond in an adaptive way to novel situations [164, 165]. These complex cognitive processes are crucial for many aspects of daily functioning, and their dysfunction plays a significant impact on academic, vocational, emotional, social, and adaptive functioning [166]. Impairment of executive functions is one of the most commonly observed deficits in schizophrenia through the various disease stages. Cognitive deficits in learning, memory, processing speed, and executive functioning are identified not only in chronic schizophrenia patients but also as early as the first episode of psychosis or even before the prodromal state [167–169]. The patients with the first psychotic episode show cognitive deficits across almost all cognitive domains, which are comparable to deficits displayed in the fully established disorder, and individuals at clinical high risk show intermittent degrees of deficits [170]. These deficits include impairment in tasks measuring conceptualization, planning, cognitive flexibility, verbal fluency, ability to solve complex problems, and working memory. The anatomical substrate associated with executive function alterations involve mostly the dorsolateral prefrontal cortex which is responsible for decision-making, and self-regulation of behavior [171]. Executive dysfunction in schizophrenia is an important clinical and social problem. Impairments in monitoring, attention shifting, planning, inhibition, rule generation, abstract thinking, and working memory, as well as the loss of skills required for the performance of complex tasks, can negatively impact patients' social and professional functioning as well as their quality of life [172].

Social cognition represents the cognitive capability to perceive, categorize and interpret social behavior of other people and concerns the various psychological processes that enable individuals to take advantage of being part of a social group. Social cognition is composed of multiple potential domains and multiple tasks can thus be used to measure it [173]. Several social cognitive subprocesses have been studied in individuals with schizophrenia, including face perception, voice perception, motor resonance, affect sharing, mentalizing, emotion experience, and emotion regulation [174]. While it is widely acknowledged that social cognition is a major determinant of functioning in schizophrenia with both direct and indirect effect, mediating neurocognition, it is less clear which domain of social cognition most strongly affect outcomes [175]. Researchers have identified four main domains of social cognition in schizophrenia: social perception, emotion processing, theory-of-mind/mentalizing, and attributional bias. Social perception refers to identifying social cues and making accurate inferences about social roles, rules, context, and relationships. Emotion processing encompasses the ability to identify and understand emotions of others and to manage emotions of oneself. Theory of mind (ToM) is the ability to reason about mental states and understand intentions, dispositions, emotions, and beliefs of both oneself and others. Attributional style/bias indicates the way in which individuals infer the causes of particular social events [176]. Studies in the field of social cognition provided growing evidence that emotion processing, mentalizing, and social perception impairments are core features of schizophrenia that are present at a comparable level in recent-onset patients, not secondary to positive symptoms or medication effects, and relatively stable over the course of illness, and detectable at attenuated levels in unaffected biological relatives of patients and in prodromal phases of the illness [177].

4.11 Other symptoms

In addition to the well-known symptoms criteria that characterized schizophrenia, there are often other symptoms that accompany psychotic episodes such as agitation, aggression, and hostility. Despite the fact that these symptoms seem alike they are considered conceptually different [178].

Agitation represents a state characterized by increased arousal with excessive motor and verbal activity, which seems very distressing to the patient. In the DSM-5, agitation is defined as a heightened motor activity linked with a feeling of inner tension [179].

On the other hand, aggression consists of an overt behavior with the intention of inflicting noxious stimulation, often with a destructive behavior, represented by verbal injuries, destroying objects, harming others, or directing aggression toward their self. Some patients that are agitated are not mandatory also aggressive, but the situation could escalate and from an agitated schizophrenic person, you could expect aggressive behavior [180]. Many studies, consider the terms violence and aggression to be the same, the difference is made only by the domains where they are used, as aggression usually appears in psychological studies or biomedical research, and violence is a term preferred by criminalists, sociologists, or police [181]. For schizophrenic patients, both of these symptoms, agitation and violent actions, represent the common reason for unvoluntary psychiatric hospitalizations, but from the population of individuals that have a diagnostic of Schizophrenia most of them are not violent, even more, they are likely to become victims than the cause of violent crimes [182]. Other studies compared the violence risk between schizophrenic patients and the general population, results found the risk to be elevated for persons with schizophrenia, actually two times higher, and an increase by nine times in patients associated with substance abuse comorbidity [183].

The last term mentioned as hostility, is a more complex symptom with a variety of meanings, including irritability, extreme suspiciously, demanding attitude, and refusal to cooperate. Specific hostility manifests during an acute phase of schizophrenia, it can be measured by the PANSS positive subscale and is usually associated with agitation [184].

4.11.1 Aggression/violence

From an interesting point of view, the link between psychotic schizophrenic patients and the symptom represented by violence is frequently discussed. There is a common question addressed to mental health clinicians regarding a patient's risk for future violence, the easement of which depends on many factors such as conditions of the evaluation, the period of time for which violent behavior is being predicted, and the most important factors would be the characteristical symptoms of schizophrenia [185]. Two of these symptoms include persecutory delusions and command auditory hallucinations, which were found in several studies as important predictors of violent behavior [186]. Nolan et al. conducted a study on schizophrenic patients with violent acts and found that more than 20% of assaults were attributed to the presence of positive symptoms [187]. More specific, false fixed beliefs of patients being followed, spied on, poisoned, threatened in some way, or the idea of losing control to an external force, such as the patient's mind being dominated by machines, or different power sources influencing him, these patients were 2 times higher at risk for engaging in aggressive actions, and even more likely predispose to violence when males were the gender evaluated [188]. In a recent study, Appelbaum et al. tried to analyze the relation between delusional content and aggression and found that the persecutory theme was significantly associated with the risk of taking action in response to the delusions [189]. Other studies pointed out, that there is an intermediate variable that links violence to delusions, and this symptom is anger that rises as a response to delusions, considered to be a key factor in this relationship [190]. The second symptom that studies referred to as being implied in the commitment of a violent act was the directive auditory hallucinations, experienced by almost half of the schizophrenic patients [191]. As a particularity, most of the command hallucinations are usually nonviolent, this is more important because researchers found out that patients are more prone to obey nonviolent commands than destructive and aggressive instructions [192]. On the other hand, a study conducted by McNeil et al. showed that from a group of 103 schizophrenic patients, a percentage of 33 reported they have had command auditory hallucinations containing instructions on how to harm people around them, but this phenomenon happened mostly during the preceding year, in general in the first years of disease evolution, and a percent of 22 of the evaluated patients actually complied with the orders given. Also, in this study authors agreed that the presence of command hallucinations, rise more than twice the risk of harming someone in the case their patients [193]. Other studies, achieved by completing a list of factors that are highly associated with the action of obeying the command hallucinations, and these include the coexistence of both delusions and auditory hallucinations, delusions that are tied to the hallucinations, that are congruent with the voices, the knowledge of the voice identity, believing that it is real, with superior power, or that it brings a benefit, not having resources in dealing with the voices, feeling out of control regarding this aspect, and the negative content of hallucinations [194–196]. In general conclusion, the majority of schizophrenic patients do not associate violent acts, but there are some data that found a greater number of total criminal convictions in patients with schizophrenia when they were matched with controls from the general population [197]. Also, patients with schizophrenia can't be characterized by the type of violence they committed; it is important to take into consideration multiple factors that have a role in this behavior [198].

4.11.2 Agitation

As mentioned earlier, agitation is a broad term, with high heterogeneity, considered more of a syndrome, with multiple causes, including Schizophrenia, defined by restlessness that can transform into excessive motor movements, often with no purpose, that has an unstable clinical course and is associated with sensible responses to internal or external stimuli [199]. The consequence of an agitation episode includes a breakthrough the therapeutic alliance, which usually is temporary and needs a fast intervention. The major risk of an agitation episode is the progression of it, which can lead to violence and also increase the hospital resources as the majority of agitated patients end up hospitalized [200]. A study estimated that 14% of an inpatients population of schizophrenia patients presented agitation, moreover the study found that approximatiely 20% of patients have episodes of agitation during their lifetime [201]. Besides the reactive agitation that can be directly connected to the content of the delusions, or triggered by the affective symptoms that accompany hallucinations, agitation in schizophrenia can appear in association with comorbid substance use or intoxication, environmental threats, or induced akathisia by the antipsychotic treatment [202]. A rare situation is the agitation of a schizophrenic patient with predominantly negative symptoms, the risk of agitation increases if the patient is noncompliant with treatment, is hospitalized many times, and presents positive symptoms [190].

Conflict of interest

The authors declare no conflict of interest.

Author details

Bianca Daniela Crecan-Suciu[1,2]* and Ramona Păunescu[1,2]

1 Department of Neurosciences, Psychiatry and Pediatric Psychiatry Chair, "Iuliu Hațieganu" University of Medicine and Pharmacy, Cluj-Napoca, Romania

2 Psychiatric Clinic, Emergency County Hospital, Cluj-Napoca, Romania

*Address all correspondence to: suciu.bianca@umfcluj.ro

References

[1] Jablensky A, Sartorius N. Is schizophrenia universal? Acta Psychiatrica Scandinavica. 1988;**78**:65-70

[2] Whitfield W. Book Reviews : The ICD-10 Classification of Mental and Behavioural Disorders: Clinical Descriptions and Diagnostic Guidelines by World Health Organization. Published by WHO, 1992, 362pp, paperback. ISBN: 92-4-154422-8. Journal of the Royal Society of Health. 1993;**113**:103-103

[3] Morel BA. Traitsé des Maladies Mentales. AJP. 1860;**17**:199-211

[4] Clouston TS. Clinical Lectures on Mental Diseases. London: J. & A. Churchill; 1904

[5] Kahlbaum KL, Berrios GE. Die Gruppirung der psychischen Krankheiten... Part III: (The classification of mental disorders ... Part III). History of Psychiatry. 1996;7:167-170

[6] Committee on State and Community Psychiatric Systems of the Council on Psychiatric Services. American Psychiatric Association. Guidelines for psychiatric practice in public sector psychiatric inpatient facilities. The American Journal of Psychiatry. 1994;**151**:797-798

[7] Jablensky A. Towards ICD–11 and DSM–V: Issues beyond 'harmonisation'. The British Journal of Psychiatry: The Journal of Mental Science. 2009;**195**:379-381

[8] Manton KG, Korten A, Woodbury MA, et al. Symptom profiles of psychiatric disorders based on graded disease classes: An illustration using data from the WHO International Pilot Study of Schizophrenia. Psychological Medicine. 1994;**24**:133-144

[9] Andreasen NC. DSM and the death of phenomenology in America: An example of unintended consequences. Schizophrenia Bulletin. 2007;**33**:108-112

[10] Sullivan PF, Kendler KS. Typology of common psychiatric syndromes. An empirical study. British Journal of Psychiatry. 1998;**173**:312-319

[11] Jurewicz I, Owen R, O'Donovan M, et al. Searching for susceptibility genes in schizophrenia. European Neuropsychopharmacology. 2001;**11**:395-398

[12] Wirt RD, Simon W. Differential Treatment and Prognosis in Schizophrenia. Springfield; Journal of Mental Science. 1959

[13] Kendell R, Jablensky A. Distinguishing between the validity and utility of psychiatric diagnoses. The American Journal of Psychiatry. 2003;**160**:4-12

[14] Andreasen NC. The validation of psychiatric diagnosis: New models and approaches. The American Journal of Psychiatry. 1995;**152**:161-162

[15] Gaebel W, Zielasek J. Schizophrenia in 2020: Trends in diagnosis and therapy. Psychiatry and Clinical Neurosciences. 2015;**69**:661-673

[16] Gaebel W, Riesbeck M, Larach VW, et al. Trends in schizophrenia diagnosis and treatment. In: Javed A, Fountoulakis KN, editors. Advances in Psychiatry. Cham: Springer International Publishing; 2019. pp. 603-619

[17] Gaebel W, Kerst A, Cyranka K. ICD-11 Mental, behavioural or neurodevelopmental disorders: Innovations and managing implementation. Archives of Psychiatry and Psychotherapy. 2019;**21**:7-12

[18] Tandon R. The nosology of schizophrenia: Toward DSM-5 and ICD-11. The Psychiatric Clinics of North America. 2012;**35**:557-569

[19] First MB, Reed GM, Hyman SE, et al. The development of the ICD-11 clinical descriptions and diagnostic guidelines for mental and behavioural disorders. World Psychiatry. 2015;**14**:82-90

[20] Reed GM, Ayuso-Mateos JL. Towards a more clinically useful International World Health Organisation classification of Mental Disorders. Revista de Psiquiatría y Salud Mental (English Edition). 2011;**4**:113-116

[21] Keller WR, Fischer BA, Carpenter WTJ. Revisiting the diagnosis of schizophrenia: Where have we been and where are we going? CNS Neuroscience & Therapeutics. 2011;**17**:83-88

[22] Mahjouri S, Lord CE. What the DSM-5 portends for research, diagnosis, and treatment of autism spectrum disorders. Current Psychiatry Reports. 2012;**14**:739-747

[23] A conceptual framework for the revision of the ICD-10 classification of mental and behavioural disorders. World Psychiatry. 2011;**10**:86-92

[24] Nordgaard J, Arnfred SM, Handest P, et al. The diagnostic status of first-rank symptoms. Schizophrenia Bulletin. 2008;**34**:137-154

[25] Gaebel W, Sartorius N, Zielasek J. Revision der Klassifikationssysteme: DSM-5 und ICD-11. Die Psychiatrie. 2018;**10**:03-04

[26] Bromet EJ, Kotov R, Fochtmann LJ, et al. Diagnostic shifts during the decade following first admission for psychosis. The American Journal of Psychiatry. 2011;**168**:1186-1194

[27] Marneros A, Rohde A, Deister A. Validity of the negative/positive dichotomy of schizophrenic disorders under long-term conditions. Psychopathology. 1995;**28**:32-37

[28] Stein DJ, Szatmari P, Gaebel W, et al. Mental, behavioral and neurodevelopmental disorders in the ICD-11: An international perspective on key changes and controversies. BMC Medicine. 2020;**18**:21

[29] Shmukler AB. The evolution of approaches to schizophrenia diagnostics: From kraepelin to ICD-11. Consortium Psychiatricum. 2021;**2**:65-70

[30] van Os J. 'Salience syndrome' replaces 'schizophrenia' in DSM-V and ICD-11: Psychiatry's evidence-based entry into the 21st century? Acta Psychiatrica Scandinavica. 2009;**120**:363-372

[31] Tandon R, Bruijnzeel D. The evolving nosology of schizophrenia: Relevance for treatment. In: Schizophrenia: Recent Advances in Diagnosis and Treatment. Psychiatric Clinics of North America. 2014. pp. 13-23

[32] Arango C, Carpenter WT. The schizophrenia construct: Symptomatic presentation. Schizophrenia Bulletin. 3rd ed2011. pp. 9-23

[33] Martinez AP, Dorahy MJ, Nesbit A, et al. Delusional beliefs and their characteristics: A comparative study between dissociative identity disorder

and schizophrenia spectrum disorders. Journal of Psychiatric Research. 2020;**131**:263-268

[34] Silva JA, Leong GB, Weinstock R. Dangerous Delusions of Misidentification of the Self. Journal of Forensic Sciences. 1995;**40**:127-138.

[35] Mueser KT, Bellack AS, Brady EU. Hallucinations in schizophrenia. Acta Psychiatrica Scandinavica. 1990;**82**:26-29

[36] Chiang Y-H, Beckstead JW, Lo S-C, et al. Association of auditory hallucination and anxiety symptoms with depressive symptoms in patients with schizophrenia: A three-month follow-up. Archives of Psychiatric Nursing. 2018;**32**:585-590

[37] Vahia VN. Diagnostic and statistical manual of mental disorders 5: A quick glance. Indian Journal of Psychiatry. 2013;**55**:220-223

[38] Lim A, Hoek HW, Deen ML, et al. Prevalence and classification of hallucinations in multiple sensory modalities in schizophrenia spectrum disorders. Schizophrenia Research. 2016;**176**:493-499

[39] Waters F, Collerton D, Ffytche DH, et al. Visual hallucinations in the psychosis spectrum and comparative information from neurodegenerative disorders and eye disease. Schizophrenia Bulletin. 2014;**40**(Suppl. 4):S233-S245

[40] Shao X, Liao Y, Gu L, et al. The etiology of auditory hallucinations in schizophrenia: From multidimensional levels. Frontiers in Neuroscience. 2021;**15**:755870

[41] Kaminski JA, Sterzer P, Mishara AL. 'Seeing Rain': Integrating phenomenological and Bayesian predictive coding approaches to visual hallucinations and self-disturbances (Ichstörungen) in schizophrenia. Consciousness and Cognition. 2019;**73**:102757

[42] Silverstein SM. Visual perception disturbances in schizophrenia: A unified model. Nebraska Symposium on Motivation. 2016;**63**:77-132

[43] Silverstein SM, Lai A. The phenomenology and neurobiology of visual distortions and hallucinations in schizophrenia: An update. Frontiers in Psychiatry. 2021;**12**:684720

[44] Keane BP, Cruz LN, Paterno D, et al. Self-reported visual perceptual abnormalities are strongly associated with core clinical features in psychotic disorders. Frontiers in Psychiatry. 2018:69-74

[45] Matthews NL, Collins KP, Thakkar KN, et al. Visuospatial imagery and working memory in schizophrenia. Cognitive Neuropsychiatry. 2014;**19**:17-35

[46] Thomas P, Mathur P, Gottesman II, et al. Correlates of hallucinations in schizophrenia: A cross-cultural evaluation. Schizophrenia Research. 2007;**92**:41-49

[47] Blom JD, Mangoenkarso E. Sexual hallucinations in schizophrenia spectrum disorders and their relation with childhood trauma. Frontiers in Psychiatry. 2018;**4**:23-34

[48] Lewandowski KE, DePaola J, Camsari GB, et al. Tactile, olfactory, and gustatory hallucinations in psychotic disorders: A descriptive study. Annals of the Academy of Medicine, Singapore. 2009;**38**:383-385

[49] Bauer SM, Schanda H, Karakula H, et al. Culture and the prevalence of hallucinations in schizophrenia.

Comprehensive Psychiatry. 2011;**52**:319-325

[50] Stevenson RJ, Langdon R, McGuire J. Olfactory hallucinations in schizophrenia and schizoaffective disorder: A phenomenological survey. Psychiatry Research. 2011;**185**:321-327

[51] Langdon R, McGuire J, Stevenson R, et al. Clinical correlates of olfactory hallucinations in schizophrenia. The British Journal of Clinical Psychology. 2011;**50**:145-163

[52] Toh WL, McCarthy-Jones S, Copolov D, et al. Have we overlooked the significance of multinodal hallucinations in schizophrenia? Psychiatry Research. 2019;**279**:358-360

[53] McCarthy-Jones S, Smailes D, Corvin A, et al. Occurrence and co-occurrence of hallucinations by modality in schizophrenia-spectrum disorders. Psychiatry Research. 2017;**252**:154-160

[54] Dudley R, Aynsworth C, Cheetham R, et al. Prevalence and characteristics of multi-modal hallucinations in people with psychosis who experience visual hallucinations. Psychiatry Research. 2018;**269**:25-30

[55] Medjkane F, Notredame C-E, Sharkey L, et al. Association between childhood trauma and multimodal early-onset hallucinations. The British Journal of Psychiatry. 2020;**216**:156-158

[56] Howard R, Rabins PV, Seeman MV, et al. Late-onset schizophrenia and very-late-onset schizophrenia-like psychosis: An international consensus. The International Late-Onset Schizophrenia Group. The American Journal of Psychiatry. 2000;**157**:172-178

[57] Melvin K, Crossley J, Cromby J. The feeling, embodiment and emotion of hallucinations in first episode psychosis: A prospective phenomenological visual-ecological study using novel multimodal unusual sensory experience (MUSE) maps. EClinicalMedicine. 2021;**41**:101153

[58] Köhler-Forsberg O, Madsen T, Behrendt-Møller I, et al. The 10-year trajectories of auditory hallucinations among 496 patients with a first schizophrenia-spectrum disorder: Findings from the OPUS cohort. Schizophrenia Research. 2022;**243**:385-391

[59] Goghari VM, Harrow M. Twenty year multi-follow-up of different types of hallucinations in schizophrenia, schizoaffective disorder, bipolar disorder, and depression. Schizophrenia Research. 2016;**176**:371-377

[60] Goghari VM, Harrow M, Grossman LS, et al. A 20-year multi-follow-up of hallucinations in schizophrenia, other psychotic, and mood disorders. Psychological Medicine. 2013;**43**:1151-1160

[61] Liddle PF. The symptoms of chronic schizophrenia. A re-examination of the positive-negative dichotomy. The British Journal of Psychiatry. 1987;**151**:145-151

[62] Toomey R, Kremen WS, Simpson JC, et al. Revisiting the factor structure for positive and negative symptoms: Evidence from a large heterogeneous group of psychiatric patients. The American Journal of Psychiatry. 1997;**154**:371-377

[63] Brekke J, Kay DD, Lee KS, et al. Biosocial pathways to functional outcome in schizophrenia. Schizophrenia Research. 2005;**80**:213-225

[64] Emsley R, Rabinowitz J, Torreman M. The factor structure for

the Positive and Negative Syndrome Scale (PANSS) in recent-onset psychosis. Schizophrenia Research. 2003;**61**:47-57

[65] Cuesta MJ, Ugarte MD, Goicoa T, et al. A taxometric analysis of schizophrenia symptoms. Psychiatry Research. 2007;**150**:245-253

[66] Evans JD, Bond GR, Meyer PS, et al. Cognitive and clinical predictors of success in vocational rehabilitation in schizophrenia. Schizophrenia Research. 2004;**70**:331-342

[67] Smith TE, Hull JW, Huppert JD, et al. Recovery from psychosis in schizophrenia and schizoaffective disorder: Symptoms and neurocognitive rate-limiters for the development of social behavior skills. Schizophrenia Research. 2002;**55**:229-237

[68] Wallwork RS, Fortgang R, Hashimoto R, et al. Searching for a consensus five-factor model of the Positive and Negative Syndrome Scale for schizophrenia. Schizophrenia Research. 2012;**137**:246-250

[69] Galderisi S, Rossi A, Rocca P, et al. The influence of illness-related variables, personal resources and context-related factors on real-life functioning of people with schizophrenia. World Psychiatry. 2014;**13**:275-287

[70] Ventura J, Thames AD, Wood RC, et al. Disorganization and reality distortion in schizophrenia: A meta-analysis of the relationship between positive symptoms and neurocognitive deficits. Schizophrenia Research. 2010;**121**:1-14

[71] Hamm JA, Renard SB, Fogley RL, et al. Metacognition and social cognition in schizophrenia: Stability and relationship to concurrent and prospective symptom assessments. Journal of Clinical Psychology. 2012;**68**:1303-1312

[72] Ventura J, Wood RC, Jimenez AM, et al. Neurocognition and symptoms identify links between facial recognition and emotion processing in schizophrenia: Meta-analytic findings. Schizophrenia Research. 2013;**151**:78-84

[73] Minor KS, Lysaker PH. Necessary, but not sufficient: Links between neurocognition, social cognition, and metacognition in schizophrenia are moderated by disorganized symptoms. Schizophrenia Research. 2014;**159**:198-204

[74] Vignapiano A, Koenig T, Mucci A, et al. Disorganization and cognitive impairment in schizophrenia: New insights from electrophysiological findings. International Journal of Psychophysiology. 2019;**145**:99-108

[75] Ortiz BB, Higuchi CH, Noto C, et al. A symptom combination predicting treatment-resistant schizophrenia—A strategy for real-world clinical practice. Schizophrenia Research. 2020;**218**:195-200

[76] Pelizza L, Leuci E, Maestri D, et al. Disorganization in first episode schizophrenia: Treatment response and psychopathological findings from the 2-year follow-up of the 'Parma Early Psychosis' program. Journal of Psychiatric Research. 2021;**141**:293-300

[77] Anderson AE, Reise SP, Marder SR, et al. Disparity between General Symptom Relief and Remission Criteria in the Positive and Negative Syndrome Scale (PANSS): A Post-treatment Bifactor Item Response Theory Model. Innovations in Clinical Neuroscience. 2017;**14**:41-53

[78] Poole JH, Ober BA, Shenaut GK, et al. Independent frontal-system deficits in schizophrenia: Cognitive, clinical,

and adaptive implications. Psychiatry Research. 1999;**85**:161-176

[79] Andreasen NC. Correlational studies of the scale for the assessment of negative symptoms and the scale for the assessment of positive symptoms: An overview and update. Psychopathology. 1995;**28**:7-17

[80] Maher BA, Manschreck TC, Linnet J, et al. Quantitative assessment of the frequency of normal associations in the utterances of schizophrenia patients and healthy controls. Schizophrenia Research. 2005;**78**:219-224

[81] Elvevåg B, Foltz PW, Weinberger DR, et al. Quantifying incoherence in speech: An automated methodology and novel application to schizophrenia. Schizophrenia Research. 2007;**93**:304-316

[82] Ruby P, Sirigu A, Decety J. Distinct areas in parietal cortex involved in long-term and short-term action planning: A PET investigation. Cortex. 2002;**38**:321-339

[83] Sitnikova T, Goff D, Kuperberg G. Neurocognitive Abnormalities During Comprehension of Real-World Goal-Directed Behaviors in Schizophrenia. Journal of Abnormal Psychology. 2009;**118**:256-277

[84] Graham Hole. Understanding intersensory integration crossmodal space and crossmodal attention.Applied Cognitive Psychology. 2005;**19**:377-378

[85] Hardy-Baylé M-C, Sarfati Y, Passerieux C. The cognitive basis of disorganization symptomatology in schizophrenia and its clinical correlates: Toward a pathogenetic approach to disorganization. Schizophrenia Bulletin. 2003;**29**:459-471

[86] Zalla T, Verlut I, Franck N, et al. Perception of dynamic action in patients with schizophrenia. Psychiatry Research. 2004;**128**:39-51

[87] Rinaldi R, Lefebvre L. Goal-directed behaviors in patients with schizophrenia: Concept relevance and updated model. Psychiatry and Clinical Neurosciences. 2016;**70**:394-404

[88] Schnell K, Heekeren K, Daumann J, et al. Correlation of passivity symptoms and dysfunctional visuomotor action monitoring in psychosis. Brain. 2008;**131**:2783-2797

[89] Blakemore SJ, Smith J, Steel R, et al. The perception of self-produced sensory stimuli in patients with auditory hallucinations and passivity experiences: Evidence for a breakdown in self-monitoring. Psychological Medicine. 2000;**30**:1131-1139

[90] Fourneret P, Franck N, Slachevsky A, et al. Self-monitoring in schizophrenia revisited. Neuroreport. 2001;**12**:1203-1208

[91] Franck N, Farrer C, Georgieff N, et al. Defective recognition of one's own actions in patients with schizophrenia. The American Journal of Psychiatry. 2001;**158**:454-459

[92] Frith CD, Blakemore S, Wolpert DM. Explaining the symptoms of schizophrenia: Abnormalities in the awareness of action. Brain Research. Brain Research Reviews. 2000;**31**:357-363

[93] Synofzik M, Vosgerau G, Voss M. The experience of agency: An interplay between prediction and postdiction. Frontiers in Psychology. 2013;**4**:127

[94] Graham-Schmidt KT, Martin-Iverson MT, Waters FAV. Self- and other-agency in people with passivity (first rank) symptoms in

schizophrenia. Schizophrenia Research. 2018;**192**:75-81

[95] Waters F, Jablensky A. Time discrimination deficits in schizophrenia patients with first-rank (passivity) symptoms. Psychiatry Research. 2009;**167**:12-20

[96] Buhusi CV, Meck WH. What makes us tick? Functional and neural mechanisms of interval timing. Nature Reviews. Neuroscience. 2005;**6**:755-765

[97] Ivry RB, Spencer RMC. The neural representation of time. Current Opinion in Neurobiology. 2004;**14**:225-232

[98] Haggard P, Clark S. Intentional action: Conscious experience and neural prediction. Consciousness and Cognition. 2003;**12**:695-707

[99] Martin B, Giersch A, Huron C, et al. Temporal event structure and timing in schizophrenia: Preserved binding in a longer 'now'. Neuropsychologia. 2013;**51**:358-371

[100] Graham KT, Martin-Iverson MT, Holmes NP, et al. Deficits in agency in schizophrenia, and additional deficits in body image, body schema, and internal timing, in passivity symptoms. Frontiers in Psychiatry. 2014;**5**:126

[101] Correll CU, Schooler NR. Negative symptoms in schizophrenia: A review and clinical guide for recognition, assessment, and treatment. Neuropsychiatric Disease and Treatment. 2020;**16**:519-534

[102] Mäkinen J, Miettunen J, Isohanni M, et al. Negative symptoms in schizophrenia: A review. Nordic Journal of Psychiatry. 2008;**62**:334-341

[103] Patel R, Jayatilleke N, Broadbent M, et al. Negative symptoms in schizophrenia: A study in a large clinical sample of patients using a novel automated method. BMJ Open. 2015;**5**:e007619

[104] Möller HJ, Jäger M, Riedel M, et al. The Munich 15-year follow-up study (MUFUSSAD) on first-hospitalized patients with schizophrenic or affective disorders: Assessing courses, types and time stability of diagnostic classification. European Psychiatry. 2011;**26**:231-243

[105] Larson MK, Walker EF, Compton MT. Early signs, diagnosis and therapeutics of the prodromal phase of schizophrenia and related psychotic disorders. Expert Review of Neurotherapeutics. 2010;**10**:1347-1359

[106] Neznanov NG, Shmukler AB, Kostyuk GP, et al. Pervyi psikhoticheskii epizod: Epidemiologicheskie aspekty organizatsii pomoshchi. Social and Clinical Psychiatry. 2018;**28**:5-11

[107] Carpenter WTJ, Heinrichs DW, Wagman AM. Deficit and nondeficit forms of schizophrenia: The concept. The American Journal of Psychiatry. 1988;**145**:578-583

[108] Buchanan RW. Persistent negative symptoms in schizophrenia: An overview. Schizophrenia Bulletin. 2007;**33**:1013-1022

[109] Kirkpatrick B, Buchanan R, Ross D, et al. A separate disease within the syndrome of schizophrenia. Archives of General Psychiatry. 2001;**58**:165-171

[110] Marder SR, Galderisi S. The current conceptualization of negative symptoms in schizophrenia. World Psychiatry. 2017;**16**:14-24

[111] Kirkpatrick B, Strauss GP, Nguyen L, et al. The brief negative symptom scale:

Psychometric properties. Schizophrenia Bulletin. 2011;**37**:300-305

[112] Blanchard JJ, Cohen AS. The structure of negative symptoms within schizophrenia: Implications for assessment. Schizophrenia Bulletin. 2006;**32**:238-245

[113] Horan WP, Kring AM, Gur RE, et al. Development and psychometric validation of the Clinical Assessment Interview for Negative Symptoms (CAINS). Schizophrenia Research. 2011;**132**:140-145

[114] Galderisi S, Mucci A, Buchanan RW, et al. Negative symptoms of schizophrenia: New developments and unanswered research questions. Lancet Psychiatry. 2018;**5**:664-677

[115] Foussias G, Agid O, Fervaha G, et al. Negative symptoms of schizophrenia: Clinical features, relevance to real world functioning and specificity versus other CNS disorders. European Neuropsychopharmacology. 2014;**24**:693-709

[116] Mosolov SN, Yaltonskaya PA. Primary and secondary negative symptoms in schizophrenia. Frontiers in Psychiatry. 2022;**12**:145-156. DOI: https://www.frontiersin.org/article/10.3389/fpsyt.2021.766692

[117] International Classification of Diseases, Eleventh Revision (ICD-11), World Health Organization (WHO) 2019/2021. Available from: https://icd.who.int/browse11

[118] Fink M, Taylor MA. The catatonia syndrome: Forgotten but not gone. Archives of General Psychiatry. 2009;**66**:1173-1177

[119] Francis A, Fink M, Appiani F, et al. Catatonia in diagnostic and statistical manual of mental disorders, fifth edition. Journal of ECT. 2010;**26**:246-247

[120] Peralta V, Campos MS, de Jalon EG, et al. DSM-IV catatonia signs and criteria in first-episode, drug-naive, psychotic patients: Psychometric validity and response to antipsychotic medication. Schizophrenia Research. 2010;**118**:168-175

[121] Rasmussen SA, Mazurek MF, Rosebush PI. Catatonia: Our current understanding of its diagnosis, treatment and pathophysiology. World Journal of Psychiatry. 2016;**6**:391-398

[122] Solmi M, Pigato GG, Roiter B, et al. Prevalence of catatonia and its moderators in clinical samples: Results from a meta-analysis and meta-regression analysis. Schizophrenia Bulletin. 2018;**44**:1133-1150

[123] Cuevas-Esteban J, Sanagustin D, Iglesias-González M. Catatonia: Back to the future of the neuropsychiatric syndrome. Medicina Clínica (Barcelona). 2022;**158**:369-377

[124] Aggarwal A, Sharma DD, Kumar R, et al. Mutism as the presenting symptom: Three case reports and selective review of literature. Indian Journal of Psychological Medicine. 2010;**32**:61-64

[125] Grover S, Naskar C, Sharma P. Treatment-resistant non-catatonic mutism in schizophrenia: A case report and review of literature. Asian Journal of Psychiatry. 2022;**71**:103067

[126] Seeman MV. Long-term non-catatonic mutism in schizophrenia: Cultural influences. Null. 2017;**10**:121-126

[127] Peralta V, Cuesta MJ. Neuromotor abnormalities in neuroleptic-naive psychotic patients: Antecedents, clinical

correlates, and prediction of treatment response. Comprehensive Psychiatry. 2011;**52**:139-145

[128] Aas M, Dazzan P, Mondelli V, et al. A systematic review of cognitive function in first-episode psychosis, including a discussion on childhood trauma, stress, and inflammation. Frontiers in Psychiatry. 2014;**4**:467-470. Available from: https://www.frontiersin.org/article/10.3389/fpsyt.2013.00182

[129] Kelleher I, Murtagh A, Clarke MC, et al. Neurocognitive performance of a community-based sample of young people at putative ultra high risk for psychosis: Support for the processing speed hypothesis. Cognitive Neuropsychiatry. 2013;**18**:9-25

[130] Grootens KP, Vermeeren L, Verkes RJ, et al. Psychomotor planning is deficient in recent-onset schizophrenia. Schizophrenia Research. 2009;**107**:294-302

[131] Morrens M, Hulstijn W, Sabbe B. Psychomotor slowing in schizophrenia. Schizophrenia Bulletin. 2007;**33**:1038-1053

[132] Walther S. Psychomotor symptoms of schizophrenia map on the cerebral motor circuit. Psychiatry Research. 2015;**233**:293-298

[133] Walther S, Strik W. Motor symptoms and schizophrenia. Neuropsychobiology. 2012;**66**:77-92

[134] Osborne KJ, Walther S, Shankman SA, et al. Psychomotor slowing in schizophrenia: Implications for endophenotype and biomarker development. Biomark Neuropsychiatry. 2020;**2**:100016

[135] Morrissette DA, Stahl SM. Affective symptoms in schizophrenia. Drug Discovery Today: Therapeutic Strategies. 2011;**8**:3-9

[136] An der Heiden W, Könnecke R, Maurer K, et al. Depression in the long-term course of schizophrenia. European Archives of Psychiatry and Clinical Neuroscience. 2005;**255**:174-184

[137] Felmet K, Zisook S, Kasckow JW. Elderly patients with schizophrenia and depression: Diagnosis and treatment. Clinical Schizophrenia & Related Psychoses. 2011;**4**:239-250

[138] Li W, Yang Y, An F-R, et al. Prevalence of comorbid depression in schizophrenia: A meta-analysis of observational studies. Journal of Affective Disorders. 2020;**273**:524-531

[139] Subsyndromal and syndromal depressive symptoms among older adults with schizophrenia spectrum disorder: Prevalence and associated factors in a multicenter study. Journal of Affective Disorders. 2019;**251**:60-70

[140] Zisook S, Nyer M, Kasckow J, et al. Depressive symptom patterns in patients with chronic schizophrenia and subsyndromal depression. Schizophrenia Research. 2006;**86**:226-233

[141] Naguy A. Depression in schizophrenia—A good or bad omen? Asia-Pacific Psychiatry. 2018;**10**:e12312

[142] Ayesa-Arriola R, Alcaraz EG, Hernández BV, et al. Suicidal behaviour in first-episode non-affective psychosis: Specific risk periods and stage-related factors. European Neuropsychopharmacology. 2015;**25**:2278-2288

[143] Li A, Huang X, Zhu T. A systematic analysis of online broadcasts of suicidality in China. Asia-Pacific Psychiatry. 2018;**10**:e12302

[144] Joseph J, Kremen WS, Franz CE, et al. Predictors of current functioning and functional decline in schizophrenia. Schizophrenia Research. 2017;**188**:158-164

[145] Alessandrini M, Lançon C, Fond G, et al. A structural equation modelling approach to explore the determinants of quality of life in schizophrenia. Schizophrenia Research. 2016;**171**:27-34

[146] Bowie CR, Harvey PD. Cognitive deficits and functional outcome in schizophrenia. Neuropsychiatric Disease and Treatment. 2006;**2**:531-536

[147] Davies G, Fowler D, Greenwood K. Metacognition as a mediating variable between neurocognition and functional outcome in first episode psychosis. Schizophrenia Bulletin. 2017;**43**:824-832

[148] Zanelli J, Mollon J, Sandin S, et al. Cognitive change in schizophrenia and other psychoses in the decade following the first episode. The American Journal of Psychiatry. 2019;**176**:811-819

[149] Alkan E, Davies G, Evans SL. Cognitive impairment in schizophrenia: Relationships with cortical thickness in fronto-temporal regions, and dissociability from symptom severity. NPJ Schizophrenia. 2021;**7**:20

[150] Bora E, Yücel M, Pantelis C. Cognitive impairment in schizophrenia and affective psychoses: Implications for DSM-V criteria and beyond. Schizophrenia Bulletin. 2010;**36**:36-42

[151] Mascio A, Stewart R, Botelle R, et al. Cognitive impairments in schizophrenia: A study in a large clinical sample using natural language processing. Frontiers In Digital Health. 2021;**3**:711941

[152] Michael GA, Dorey J-M, Rey R, et al. Attention in schizophrenia: Impaired inhibitory control, faulty attentional resources, or both? Psychiatry Research. 2020;**290**:113164

[153] Alan B. Working memory. Science. 1992;**255**:556-559

[154] Lee J, Park S. Working memory impairments in schizophrenia: A meta-analysis. Journal of Abnormal Psychology. 2005;**114**:599-611

[155] Forbes NF, Carrick LA, McIntosh AM, et al. Working memory in schizophrenia: A meta-analysis. Psychological Medicine. 2009;**39**:889-905

[156] Dienel SJ, Schoonover KE, Lewis DA. Cognitive dysfunction and prefrontal cortical circuit alterations in schizophrenia: Developmental trajectories. Biological Psychiatry. 2022;**92**:450-459. DOI: 10.1016/j.biopsych.2022.03.002

[157] Smucny J, Dienel SJ, Lewis DA, et al. Mechanisms underlying dorsolateral prefrontal cortex contributions to cognitive dysfunction in schizophrenia. Neuropsychopharmacology. 2022;**47**:292-308

[158] Park S, Gooding DC. Working memory impairment as an endophenotypic marker of a schizophrenia diathesis. Schizophrenia Research: Cognition. 2014;**1**:127-136

[159] Tulving E. Episodic memory: From mind to brain. Annual Review of Psychology. 2002;**53**:1-25

[160] Kwok SC, Xu X, Duan W, et al. Autobiographical and episodic memory deficits in schizophrenia: A narrative review and proposed agenda for research. Clinical Psychology Review. 2021;**83**:101956

[161] Ranganath C, Minzenberg MJ, Ragland JD. The cognitive neuroscience

of memory function and dysfunction in schizophrenia. Biological Psychiatry. 2008;**64**:18-25

[162] İmamoğlu A, Foubert C, Healey MK, et al. Episodic memory impairment in children and adolescents at risk for schizophrenia: A role for context processing. Schizophrenia Research: Cognition. 2022;**28**:100241

[163] Kraguljac N, Srivastava A, Lahti A. Memory deficits in schizophrenia: A selective review of functional magnetic resonance imaging (fMRI) studies. Behavioral Sciences (Basel, Switzerland). 2013;**3**:330-347

[164] Diamond A. Executive functions. Annual Review of Psychology. 2013;**64**:135-168

[165] Zelazo P, Craik F, Booth L. Executive function across the life span. Acta Psychologica. 2004;**115**:167-183

[166] Hunter SJ, Sparrow EP, editors. Executive Function and Dysfunction: Identification, Assessment and Treatment. Cambridge: Cambridge University Press. Epub ahead of print; 2012. DOI: 10.1017/CBO9780511977954

[167] Raffard S, Bayard S. Understanding the executive functioning heterogeneity in schizophrenia. Brain and Cognition. 2012;**79**:60-69

[168] Freedman D, Brown A. The developmental course of executive functioning in schizophrenia. International Journal of Developmental Neuroscience: The Official Journal of the International Society for Developmental Neuroscience. 2010;**29**:237-243

[169] Bora E, Murray RM. Meta-analysis of cognitive deficits in ultra-high risk to psychosis and first-episode psychosis: Do the cognitive deficits progress over, or after, the onset of psychosis? Schizophrenia Bulletin. 2014;**40**:744-755

[170] Hwang WJ, Lee TY, Shin W-G, et al. Global and specific profiles of executive functioning in prodromal and early psychosis. Frontiers in Psychiatry. 2019;**10**:89-92. Available from: https://www.frontiersin.org/article/10.3389/fpsyt.2019.00356

[171] Orellana G, Slachevsky A. Executive functioning in schizophrenia. Frontiers in Psychiatry. 2013;**4**:12-15

[172] Tyburski E, Mak M, Sokołowski A, et al. Executive dysfunctions in schizophrenia: A critical review of traditional, ecological, and virtual reality assessments. Journal of Clinical Medicine; 10. Epub ahead of print 24 June 2021. DOI: 10.3390/jcm10132782.

[173] Harvey PD, Bosia M, Cavallaro R, et al. Cognitive dysfunction in schizophrenia: An expert group paper on the current state of the art. Schizophrenia Research: Cognition. 2022;**29**:100249

[174] Green MF, Horan WP, Lee J. Social cognition in schizophrenia. Nature Reviews. Neuroscience. 2015;**16**:620-631

[175] Bechi M, Spangaro M. Chapter four—Impact of social cognitive deficits on community functioning. In: Lewandowski KE, Moustafa AA, editors. Social Cognition in Psychosis. Amsterdam: Academic Press; pp. 89-123

[176] Weinreb S, Li F, Kurtz MM. A meta-analysis of social cognitive deficits in schizophrenia: Does world region matter? Schizophrenia Research. 2022;**243**:206-213

[177] Green M, Horan W, Lee J. Nonsocial and social cognition in schizophrenia: Current evidence and future directions. World Psychiatry. 2019;**18**:146-161

[178] Powell G, Caan W, Crowe M. What events precede violent incidents in psychiatric hospitals? The British Journal of Psychiatry. 1994;**165**:107-112

[179] Fagiolini A. Appropriate treatments for agitation associated with schizophrenia: Control of acute agitation and maintenance of efficacy. European Psychiatry. 2007;**22**:S89-S90

[180] Volicer L, Citrome L, Volavka J. Measurement of agitation and aggression in adult and aged neuropsychiatric patients: Review of definitions and frequently used measurement scales. CNS Spectrums. 2017;**22**:407-414

[181] Cho D, Lindenmayer J. Aripiprazole-induced agitation after clozapine discontinuation. The Journal of Clinical Psychiatry. 2009;**70**:141-143

[182] Fazel S, Grann M. The population impact of severe mental illness on violent crime. The American Journal of Psychiatry. 2006;**163**:1397-1403

[183] Fazel S, Gulati G, Linsell L, et al. Schizophrenia and violence: Systematic review and meta-analysis. PLoS Medicine. 2009;**6**:e1000120

[184] Buss AH, Durkee A. An inventory for assessing different kinds of hostility. Journal of Consulting Psychology. 1957;**21**:343-349

[185] Douglas KS, Guy LS, Hart SD. Psychosis as a risk factor for violence to others: A meta-analysis. Psychological Bulletin. 2009;**135**:679-706

[186] Witt K, van Dorn R, Fazel S. Risk factors for violence in psychosis: Systematic review and meta-regression analysis of 110 studies. PLoS One. 2013;**8**:e55942

[187] Nolan KA, Czobor P, Roy BB, et al. Characteristics of assaultive behavior among psychiatric inpatients. Psychiatric Services. 2003;**54**:1012-1016

[188] Buchanan A, Reed A, Wessely S, et al. Acting on delusions. II: The phenomenological correlates of acting on delusions. The British Journal of Psychiatry: The Journal of Mental Science. 1993;**163**:77-81

[189] Appelbaum PS, Robbins PC, Vesselinov R. Persistence and stability of delusions over time. Comprehensive Psychiatry. 2004;**45**:317-324

[190] Coid JW, Ullrich S, Kallis C, et al. The relationship between delusions and violence: Findings from the east London first episode psychosis study. JAMA Psychiatry. 2013;**70**:465-471

[191] Shawyer F, MacKinnon A, Farhall J, et al. Command hallucinations and violence: Implications for detention and treatment. Psychiatry, Psychology and Law. 2003;**10**:97-107

[192] Hacker D, Birchwood M, Tudway J, et al. Acting on voices: Omnipotence, sources of threat, and safety-seeking behaviours. The British Journal of Clinical Psychology. 2008;**47**:201-213

[193] McNiel DE, Eisner JP, Binder RL. The relationship between command hallucinations and violence. Psychiatric Services. 2000;**51**:1288-1292

[194] Erkwoh R, Willmes K, Eming-Erdmann A, et al. Command hallucinations: Who obeys and who resists when? Psychopathology. 2002;**35**:272-279

[195] Bucci S, Birchwood M, Twist L, et al. Predicting compliance with command hallucinations: Anger, impulsivity and appraisals of voices' power and intent. Schizophrenia Research. 2013;**147**:163-168

[196] Fox JR, Gray NS, Lewis H. Factors determining compliance with command hallucinations with violent content: The role of social rank, perceived power of the voice and voice malevolence. Null. 2004;**15**:511-531

[197] Wallace C, Mullen PE, Burgess P. Criminal offending in schizophrenia over a 25-year period marked by deinstitutionalization and increasing prevalence of comorbid substance use disorders. The American Journal of Psychiatry. 2004;**161**:716-727

[198] Dodge KA, Lochman JE, Harnish JD, et al. Reactive and proactive aggression in school children and psychiatrically impaired chronically assaultive youth. Journal of Abnormal Psychology. 1997;**106**:37-51

[199] Garriga M, Pacchiarotti I, Hidalgo D, et al. Detection and management of agitation in psychiatry: A Delphi expert consensus study. European Psychiatry. 2016;**33**:S170-S170

[200] Zeller SL, Rhoades RW. Systematic reviews of assessment measures and pharmacologic treatments for agitation. Clinical Therapeutics. 2010;**32**:403-425

[201] Soyka M. Aggression in schizophrenia: Assessment and prevalence. British Journal of Psychiatry. 2002;**180**:278-279

[202] Citrome L, Krakowski M, Greenberg WM, et al. Antiaggressive effect of quetiapine in a patient with schizoaffective disorder. The Journal of Clinical Psychiatry. 2001;**62**:901

Section 3

Clinical Intervention

Chapter 3

Nursing Care for Schizophrenic Clients: Recent Advances and Client-Centred Nursing Care Perspectives

Ek-Uma Imkome

Abstract

Schizophrenia is one of the leading causes of disability worldwide; psychiatric disorders can result in impairments of perception, poor self-care, and decreased performance in activities of daily living. Treatment and nursing care are vital options for clients to improve their signs and symptoms, especially during the COVID-19 pandemic. The planning of nursing care for individual schizophrenic clients is essential and will help them have a satisfactory quality of life. Current nursing should be provided according to the client's needs and particular problems, such as the presence of comorbidities, amidst the state quarantine. The current nursing care focuses on telenursing, with nurses implementing information technology to provide the necessary care. Despite the physical distancing, clients can access nursing services efficiently, with nurses being flexible enough to continue their care provision during the COVID-19 pandemic.

Keywords: schizophrenia, telenursing, nursing care, client-centered, psychiatric disorder

1. Introduction

The most common impairments of schizophrenic patients include delusions, illusions, hallucinations, anger, hostility, and aggression. Nursing care for this population should focus on patient-centered needs and individual problems. In addition, during the coronavirus pandemic, telenursing should be provided to prevent infection and adhere to social distancing rules. The practical nursing process application will reflect the effective nursing outcomes.

When the global coronavirus SARS-CoV-2 (COVID-19) epidemic hit, nursing care was pressed to switch to telenursing. Telenursing is primarily performed by the nurses using a cell phone, computer, audio and video technology, or advanced digital and optical communications, in order to deliver health care and provide remote, synchronous (e.g., via live interactive videoconference) or asynchronous (e.g., the information is stored electronically) care. This type of health care usually falls within care management for emergent situations, coordination of care, and health maintenance services. It is considered beneficial for both the patient and nurse; the patient benefits from increased access to health care services, while the nurse benefits from a more flexible and less physically stressful work environment.

Telenursing is increasingly prevalent in the nursing domain because of a preoccupation with cutting down on health care costs, an increase in the number of aging and chronically ill individuals, and a rise in the coverage of health care to distant, rural, minor, or sparsely populated regions. Telenursing, providing nursing care at a distance using new technologies, is identified as one alternative. Among its many benefits, telenursing may help prevent a shortage of nurses, reduce distance and save travel time, and keep patients out of the hospital. A greater degree of job satisfaction has also been registered among telenurses.

Telenursing has been considered a potential solution to service delivery challenges during the COVID-19 pandemic, mainly due to its compliance with physical distancing measures and stay-at-home orders implemented by several governments to curb the spread of infection. Additionally, telenursing is benefit for the nurse to providing telenursing care for victims in disasters in a simulated study for introducing of possibility nursing interventions, telenursing education on nurses' compliance with standard precautions during the COVID-19 pandemic [1], telenursing training based on family-centered empowerment pattern on compliance with diet regimen in patients with diabetes mellitus, education through telenursing can increase the quality of life of COVID-19 patients [2], telenursing in COVID-19 times and maternal health: whatsapp® as a support tool, telenursing on attachment and stress in mothers of preterm infants, telephone-based telenursing on perceived stressors among older adults receiving hemodialysis, telenursing on levels of depression and anxiety in caregivers of patients with stroke, Treatment of Obesity Among Youth With Intellectual and Developmental Disabilities: An Emerging Role for Telenursing [3], Telenursing intervention increases psychiatric medication adherence in schizophrenia outpatients [4]. Telenursing are ongoing to increase both nationally and internationally. A primary role of telenursing is to channel clients towards appropriate levels of nursing care thereby reducing healthcare costs and freeing up resources [5, 6].

The purpose of this chapter is two-fold. First, it describes the principle of caring for a person with schizophrenia during the COVID-19 pandemic. Second, it aims to describe the processes behind understanding the facilitators and barriers to telenursing during the pandemic.

The principle of caring for a person with schizophrenia during the COVID-19 pandemic.

This chapter provides an overview of telenursing and its application to nurses' daily practical challenges. The principle of caring for a person with schizophrenia during the COVID-19 pandemic is as below:

2. Cognitive and perceptive disorders (delusions, illusions, and hallucinations)

2.1 Delusions

A delusion refers to a fixed false belief with no basis in reality in the psychotic phase of an illness. A common characteristic of schizophrenic delusions includes the direct, immediate, and total certainty with which the client holds these beliefs. A person with schizophrenia is probably suspicious, mistrustful, and guarded about disclosing personal information. They may examine a room periodically or speak in hushed, secretive tones due to delusions.

2.2 Illusions

An illusion distorts one's senses by misinterpreting true sensory stimuli, as in visual illusions. Some misconceptions are based on general assumptions that the brain makes by using organizational principles, the client's perceptual ability and motion perception, and perceptual dependability. The causes of illusions are biological, psychological, and physical. For example, hearing voices regardless of the background would be a hallucination, whereas hearing voices instead of the sound of running water would be an illusion; individuals watching a ventriloquist will perceive that the voice is coming from the dummy since they can see the dummy's mouth moving (**Table 1**).

2.3 Applying the nursing process for clients with delusion

2.3.1 Nursing diagnosis

Risk for self-harm/other harmful activities related to disturbed thought processes

Types of delusions	Description
Persecutory delusions	The conviction of a person with schizophrenia regarding others wanting to harm, spy on, follow, ridicule, or belittle them. Sometimes, they cannot name who these "others" are. They may think that their food has been poisoned, and their bedroom has been bugged with listening devices. Occasionally, specific individuals, including family members, may be named as the "persecutor." Sometimes, the "persecutor" is the government, the Federal Bureau of Investigation, or any other powerful organization.
Grandiose delusions	The client believes that they are famous or capable of incredible feats. ***Examples:*** The client may claim to be engaged to a famous movie star or related to some public figure, such as claiming to be the daughter of the president of the United States, or they may claim to have found a cure for cancer.
Religious delusions	The client believes that they center around the second coming of Christ or another significant religious figure or prophet. These religious delusions appear suddenly as part of the client's psychosis and are not part of their or others' religious faith. ***Examples:*** The client claims to be the Messiah or some prophet sent from God; they believe that God communicates directly with them, or they have an extraordinary religious task or special spiritual powers.
Somatic delusions	They believe that they have an illness, but it is not valid. Even though they are healthy, it does not change these beliefs. ***Examples:*** A male client may say he is pregnant, or a client may report having decaying intestines or worms in the brain.
Delusions of reference	The conviction of a person with schizophrenia about television broadcasts, music, or newspaper articles has a special meaning for them. ***Examples:*** The client may report that the president was speaking directly to them on a news broadcast or sent particular messages through newspaper articles.

Table 1.
Five types of delusions.

2.3.2 Assessment data

- Thinking not based on reality
- Disorientation
- Labile affect
- Short attention span
- Impaired judgment
- Distractibility

2.3.3 Goals

- Build a relationship with the client based on empathy and trust.
- Encourage an understanding of the features and appropriate management of delusions.
- Promote coping strategies.
- Promote medication compliance and healthy lifestyle choices (diet, exercise, no smoking, and substance abuse).
- Promote social skills and support networks.
- Promote effective working relationships and communication.

2.3.4 Outcomes

Immediate: The client will

- Experience safety
- Have decreased anxiety levels
- Respond to reality-based interactions

Stabilization: The client will

- Respond to reality-based interactions
- Have increased concentration to complete tasks

Community: The client will

- Verbalize recognition of delusional thoughts
- Experience safety (**Table 2**)

Nursing interventions (* Apply telenursing)	Rationale
Assessment of the level of • Thinking not based on reality • Disorientation • Labile affect • Short attention span • Impaired judgment • Distractibility	To plan for the care of specific symptoms.
Communicating with sincerity and honesty.*	The person with schizophrenia and delusions is susceptible to others and can recognize insincerity. Evasive comments or hesitation reinforce mistrust.
Be consistent in setting expectations, rules, and so forth.	May decrease anxiety, which leads to severe delusion.
Do not make promises that you cannot keep.	Broken promises lead to the client's mistrust of others.
Encourage the client to start small talk with another client.	To promote social skills.
Formulating procedures and ensuring the client understands the procedures before providing nursing care.	When clients have full knowledge of the procedures, they are more likely to feel safe and have no anxiety.
Give positive feedback.	Positive feedback for genuine success enhances them to maintain positive behavior.
Use unconditional positive regard.	Recognizing the client's perceptions can help nurses understand their feelings and provide more chances to talk with them to know about their needs.
Avoid vague or evasive remarks and do not convince the client that their delusions are false or unreal.	An argument can interfere with the development of trust.
Interact with the client based on the present reality technique.	Interacting with reality can enhance the perception of the client's actual situation.
Promote one-on-one activities, then in small groups, and gradually in larger groups for the person with schizophrenia.	A suspicious client can best deal with one person at first. The steady introduction of others is enforced as the client tolerates less hostility.
Support the client's accomplishments, such as completing projects, tasks fulfilled and initiating interactions.	Recognizing the client's accomplishments can decrease anxiety and promote self-esteem.
Use empathy regarding the client's feelings; reassure the client of your presence and recognition. *	Empathy conveys your caring, interest, and acceptance of the client.
Avoid being judgmental, belittling, or joking about the client's beliefs.	The client may not appreciate or feel rejected by attempts at humor.
Directly interject doubt about delusions when the client is ready to accept, with this sentence, "I find that hard to believe." Avoid disagreeing but give information about the actual situation as you see it.	Once the client trusts you, they may become willing to doubt the delusion if you express your doubt.
Ask the client if they can see that the delusions interfere with or cause problems in their lives.	The question may help the nurse in planning care and can decrease the client's anxiety from delusion
Provide medication as a prescription and educate them about the drug and positive benefits of medication adherence [7].	The medication will balance neurotransmitters and decrease psychotic symptoms, such as delusions.

Nursing interventions (* Apply telenursing)	Rationale
Record vital signs and monitor medication-induced movement disorders and adverse effects.	To record signs and symptoms during medication treatment and plan a client-centered nursing intervention.
Provide cognitive compensatory interventions and cognitive remediation according to the client's needs [8].	Cognitive compensatory interventions aim to ease psychosocial disability by targeting straight-line functioning using aids and strategies, thereby minimizing cognitive impairment.
Encourage clients to join the group of internal self-management strategies, such as self-talk during task completion, paraphrasing instructions, and using mental imagery [9–11]	Internal self-management strategies facilitate more efficient cognitive processing during task performance regarding categorical relationships to aid memory.

Table 2.
Nursing interventions.

2.4 Sensorium and intellectual processes: Hallucinations

The main psychotic symptom of people with schizophrenia is hallucinations. A hallucination refers to false sensory perceptions that appear real. Hallucinations are related to five senses and bodily sensations. They can be both threatening and pleasant (**Table 3**).

In psychotic episodes, disorientation of time and place, as well as depersonalization, are common in Cl. Although clients can state their name correctly, they think that their body belongs to someone else or that their spirit is separated from the body. They may also demonstrate poor intellectual functioning. The client cannot pay sufficient attention to display their academic abilities accurately. The nurse is more likely to obtain accurate assessments of the client's intellectual abilities when their thought

Types	Description
Auditory hallucinations	These comprise voices demanding that the client take action, often to harm the self or others, and are considered dangerous. The most common type involves hearing sounds, most often voices, talking to or about the client. There may be one or multiple agents; a familiar or unfamiliar person's voice may be speaking.
Visual hallucinations	They comprise visual images that do not exist at all.
Olfactory hallucinations	These involve a specific olfactory sense that smells something wrong, such as urine, feces, or the body.
Tactile hallucinations	Tactile hallucinations are most frequently found in clients undergoing alcohol withdrawal; they rarely occur in clients with schizophrenia. The client will feel like a bug on their skin and try to eliminate it.
Gustatory hallucinations	These hallucinations feel like a client's taste is lingering in the mouth or the fact that food tastes like something else. The taste may be metallic, bitter, or represented as a specific taste.
Synesthetic hallucinations	The client reports feeling like bodily functions are usually unnoticeable. Examples would be the sensation of urine forming or impulses being transmitted through the brain.
Kinaesthetic hallucinations	The client is immobile but reports the sensation of bodily movement. Physical activity is odd, such as floating.

Table 3.
Types of hallucinations [12].

processes are more transparent. They often have obscurity with abstract thinking and may respond literally to other public situations and the environment.

2.5 Applying the nursing process for clients with hallucinations

2.5.1 Nursing diagnosis

Change in the amount or patterns of incoming stimuli accompanied by a diminished, exaggerated, distorted, or impaired response to such stimuli related to disturbed sensory perception

2.5.2 Related factors

- Altered sensory perception.
- Altered sensory reception: transmission or integration.
- Neurological/biochemical changes/stress.

2.5.3 Defining characteristics

- It has altered communication patterns.
- Hallucinations/auditory distortions/disorientation to person/place/time.
- Change in problem-solving patterns.
- Frequent blinking of the eyes and grimacing/inappropriate responses.
- Mumbling to self, talking or laughing/tilting the head as if listening to someone.
- A reported or measured change in sensory acuity.

2.5.4 Desired outcomes

The clients will

- State the symptoms they recognize when their stress levels are high.
- State that the voices are no longer intimidating, nor do they obstruct their life.
- State, using a scale from 1–10, that "the voices" are less frequent and intimidating when aided by medication and nursing care.
- Maintain role performance and social relationships/monitor their intensity of anxiety.
- Identify the stressful life events that trigger hallucinations, and personal interventions that decrease or lower the intensity or frequency of hallucinations (e.g., listening to music, wearing headphones, reading aloud, jogging, socializing).

- Demonstrate a stress reduction technique that distracts them from the voices (**Table 4**).

2.6 Conclusion

There is a variety of nursing care that can be provided for a person with cognitive impairment, such as schizophrenic clients in the schizophrenia disorder spectrum. Holistic care is always the go-to approach for decreasing the negative signs and symptoms. Psychosocial and compensatory interventions for cognitive impairment in psychotic disorders are famous and influential in improving functioning as well as decreasing the negative and general symptoms. Continuous compensatory interventions are associated with more significant improvements in functioning. Additionally, medication adherence, social function, and social support are critical factors that nurses should be concerned about, training the clients and caregivers accordingly.

3. Behavioural problems (anger, hostility, and aggression)

Anger, hostility, and aggression are common behavioral problems in schizophrenic clients. When handled appropriately and expressed assertively, anger can be a positive force that helps resolve conflicts, solve problems, and make decisions; anger results from a person being frustrated, hurt, or afraid. Anger energizes the body physically for self-defense by activating the "fight-or-flight" response mechanism. However, it can cause physical or emotional problems and interfere with relationships when expressed inappropriately or suppressed. Anger is perceived as a negative feeling. People who are uncomfortable reveal their anger directly. However, anger can be a normal response when situations are inequitable or undue, personal rights are not respected, or realistic expectations are not met. If the person can express their anger energetically, problem-solving or conflict resolution is possible. Anger becomes negative when someone rejects or suppresses it if they are uncomfortable expressing it. Examples of the consequences of anger include migraine, headaches, ulcers, coronary artery disease, depression, and low self-esteem.

Inappropriately expressed anger can lead to hostility and aggression. Some people express their angry feelings through safe activities, such as hitting a punching bag or yelling. Such actions, called catharsis, are supposed to provide a release for anger. However, catharsis can increase rather than alleviate anger. Practical methods of anger expression, such as assertive communication, should replace angry, aggressive outbursts of temper, such as yelling or throwing things. Controlling one's temper or managing anger effectively should not be confused with suppressing angry feelings, leading to the problems described earlier.

3.1 Hostility and aggression

Hostility, also called verbal assault, is an emotion expressed through negative verbal outbursts, uncooperative rules or norms, or hostile behavior. It occurs when individuals feel threatened or have no power. Hostile behavior causes emotional harm and leads to physical aggression. Verbal and physical aggression is meant to harm another person to experience fulfillment, caused by delusions and/or hallucinations in the schizophrenia spectrum. Some clients with psychiatric disorders display hostile or physically aggressive behavior that challenges the professional nurses.

Nursing interventions (* Apply telenursing)	Rationale
Assessment of the level of: • Altered sensory perception. • Altered sensory reception: transmission or integration. • Biochemical factors, such as those manifested by an inability to concentrate. • Chemical alterations (e.g., medications, electrolyte imbalances). • Neurological/biochemical changes/psychological stress. Or use the scale to screen the sign and symptoms [13].	To assess the client's needs and problems and plan for nursing intervention.
Give details and accept that you do not hear the voices using the present reality technique. *	Validating that your truth does not include voices can help the client cast "doubt" on the validity of their voices.
Monitor signs of increasing fear, anxiety, or agitation.*	Fear, anxiety, or agitation is the warning sign of hallucinations and can decrease them.
Explore how the client experiences the hallucinations, such as content, frequency, influencing factors, and coping with delusion [7].	Exploring the hallucinations and sharing the experience can help give the person a sense of power that they might be able to manage the hallucinatory voices.
Help the client to identify the needs that might underlie the hallucination. In what other ways can these needs be met.	Hallucinations might reflect the need for anger, power, self-esteem, and sexuality.
Help the client recognize times when the hallucinations are most rife and fearsome.	The helps both the nurse and client to recognize the situations and times that might be most anxiety-provoking and intimidating.
Provide environmental precautions when the delusion or hallucination commands them to harm the self. • Notify the health care team and administration according to unit protocol. • Document what the client says, and if they are a threat to others, document who was contacted and notified (use agency protocol as a guide).	People often obey hallucinatory commands to kill themselves or others. Early assessment and intervention might save lives.
When clients start to hallucinate, stay with them and tell the voices they "hear" to go away. Repeat often in a matter-of-fact manner.	The client can sometimes learn to push voices aside when given repeated instructions, especially within a trusting relationship.
Decrease environmental stimuli when possible (low noise, minimal activity).	Decrease the potential for anxiety that might trigger hallucinations. This helps calm the client down.
Intervene through one-on-one interaction, seclusion, or PRN medication (as ordered) when appropriate.	Use chemical or physical restraints following unit protocols in case of uncontrol.
Keep to simple, essential, reality-based topics of talk and support the client in focusing on one thought at a time.	The client's thoughts might be confused and muddled; this caring helps the client focus on and comprehend reality-based issues.
Find which activities can reduce anxiety and distract the client from a hallucination, and perform training with the client, such as relaxation techniques [14].	Anxiety and stress lead to hallucinations, and relaxation techniques can reduce stress and anxiety, which will decrease hallucination.
Keep clients in reality-based activities, such as group activities.	Redirecting the client's energy to acceptable activities can decrease and distract them from hallucinations.
Provide flexible services, such as tele counseling and medication delivery.*	This would support the client in receiving continuous treatment.

Table 4.
Nursing interventions and rationale.

Phase of aggression	Description	Behavioral expression
Triggering phase	A situation initiates the client's expression of anger/ hostility.	Restlessness, anxiety, tetchiness, pacing, muscle tension, tachypnoea, speaking loudly, anger.
Escalation phase	Loss of control.	Pale or flushed face, yelling, swearing, being agitated, threatening, demanding, having clenched fists, threatening gestures, hostility, loss of ability to solve the problem or think clearly.
Crisis phase	Loss of control.	Loss of emotional and physical control, throwing objects, kicking, hitting, spitting, biting, scratching, shrieking, screaming, and poor communication.
Recovery phase	Regains physical and emotional control.	Lowering the tone of voice; decreased power tension; clearer, more rational message; bodily relaxation
Post-crisis	Reconciliation with others proceeds to the execution level before the aggressive occurrence and its antecedents.	Regret, apologies, crying, calming down, separation

Table 5.
Five-phase aggression cycle [15].

Hostile and aggressive behavior can be sudden and unexpected. Clients with psychotic illnesses are much more likely to harm themselves than others. In contrast, clients with paranoid delusions may believe others are out to get them, assuming they are protecting themselves; they retaliate with aggression or hostility. Some clients have auditory hallucinations that dominate them to hurt others. Overall, violent clients are more symptomatic, have poorer functioning, and lack insight. Some clients with depression have anger attacks. These sudden intense spells of anger typically occur in situations where the depressed person feels emotionally trapped. Anger attacks engage verbal expressions of anger or rage but no physical aggression. Clients identify these anger attacks as uncharacteristic behavior unsuitable for the situation. The anger in some depressed clients is related to irritable mood, overreaction to minor annoyances, and decreased coping abilities (**Table 5**).

3.2 Application of the nursing process

3.2.1 Nursing diagnoses

The risk for other-directed forms of violence related to ineffective coping

Risk factors	
• Potential violence • Destruction of property • Homicidal/suicidal ideation • Harm to self or others • Assaultive behavior • Neurologically disordered • Substance abuse	• Agitation or restlessness • Out of control • Psychotic symptoms (delusions/ hallucinations) • Personality disorder/ conduct disorder • Manic episode • Posttraumatic stress disorder (PTSD)

3.2.2 Expected outcomes

Immediate: The client will

- Be free of self-harm.
- Decrease violence/aggressive behavior

Stabilization: The client will

- Demonstrate the ability to exercise internal control over their behavior.
- Show no psychotic behavior.
- Identify strategies to deal with tension and aggressive feelings in a non-destructive manner.
- State feelings of anxiety, fear, anger, or hostility verbally or in a non-destructive manner.
- Express an understanding of aggressive behavior, associated disorder(s), and medications, if any.

Community: The client will

- Contribute to treatment-associated psychiatric problems.
- Show internal control of behavior when faced with stress (**Table 6**).

3.3 The facilitators and barriers to telenursing during the pandemic

Nurses play a pivotal role in the provision of mental and physical healthcare. Telenursing, the use of information and communication technologies to deliver and support healthcare directly to the setting, is emerging as an essential application for nurses. The empirical evidence supports its use in specific areas and guides those thinking of implementing telehealth in their practice. The future of home telehealth lies in carefully considered and designed research, ongoing education and training, and a multidisciplinary approach. This chapter aims to stimulate the consideration of home telehealth as an application that may improve nursing care and patient outcomes.

There is massive potential for technology such as telenursing to transform people's experience, including assisting with chronic disease management, coordinated care, and guided self-care for consumers. Innovative technologies are increasingly available to assist in maintaining health and independent living.

The beginning of 2020 has been characterized by the pandemic outbreak of a novel human Coronavirus named SARS-Cov-2. This virus is responsible for causing a disease, COVID-19, that often causes only mild illness but can also make some people very ill. More rarely, the disease can be fatal, especially among older people and those with pre-existing medical conditions who spread the virus.

That allowed to contain the spread of the virus, helping the health system to face the demands of thousands of people needing hospital advanced care. On the other hand, it resulted in worse health among people not affected by the virus. Recently, a review investigated the relationships between telenursing and health. The authors identified health problems (musculoskeletal problems, psychological problems, overwork, and others) and benefits (stress reduction, greater flexibility, better work-life balance/control, and enhanced job satisfaction).

At the end of March 2020, Italy was the world's most affected country by the novel coronavirus spread. The advanced average age of the population, together with a particular social structure, has also contributed to making the death rate of this country among the highest in the world.

The pandemic forced Governments to establish lockdown measures such as the closing of schools, universities, banks, parks, supermarkets, and non-essential businesses, limiting movements and transport, and promoting social distancing, to slow down the and a lower risk of burnout but on the other hand, the responders think that working from home diminishes their promotion opportunities and weakens ties with their colleagues and employer

Integrating technology into health care has created both advantages and disadvantages for patients, providers, and healthcare systems alike. Overall, the benefits of technology in health care outweigh the risks; however, proper measures must be taken to ensure successful implementation and integration. Accuracy, validity, confidentiality, and privacy of health data and information are key issues that must be addressed for successful technology implementation. This chapter examines the risks and benefits of technology in health care, the availability of health information online, and how technology affects relationships within the healthcare setting.

3.4 The advantage of telenursing during the pandemic

The COVID-19 pandemic has forced most countries to implement social distancing measures, also known as "lockdown," to reduce the virus transmission through respiratory droplets and contact routes by increasing physical distance or social distance aggregations19. The adoption and development of telenursing helped reduce some of the consequences of the current health crisis on the economy. It allowed continuing business even if workplaces were inaccessible, and telenursing has a significant emotional impact on nurses and patients, with the appearance of negative emotions such as loneliness, irritation, worry, and guilt. Telenursing overall was also found to experience more mental health support than usual care. The correlation may have been influenced by the current pandemic situation, which can feel that receiving information from nurses via telephone can be much safer than going to the hospital and taking public transport. People with lower educational levels had a lower risk of psychological distress than those with higher education. That assumption contrasts with solid evidence that low socioeconomic position is often associated with severe mental health disorders, such as depression.

What emerged about lifestyle habits is the rise of unhealthy behaviors among the responders who reported higher levels of psychological distress and lowered perceived well-being. Half of the responders reported to be smokers have increased the number of daily cigarettes during the lockdown. Tobacco smoking is a well-known coping strategy against psychological stress 26. Many studies 27,29 have also reported that those who smoke or drink alcohol usually increase their consumption in stressful conditions. Eating habits changed for almost half of the participants, and most of them

Implementation (* Apply telenursing)	Rationale
Build a trusting relationship and keep calm.	Trust can reduce the client's fears and aid effective communication. Your behavior provides a role model for the client and communicates that you can and will provide control.
The nurse should be assessing: 1. Risk factors that influence aggression in the psychiatric environment. 2. A history of violent or aggressive behavior. 3. Determination of how the client with a history of aggression handles anger and what the client believes is helpful in assisting them in controlling or non-aggressively managing angry feelings. Clients who are angry and frustrated and think that no one is listening to them are more prone to behave hostile or aggressive. 4. History a. Violence b. A history of being personally victimized c. Substance abuse 5. Which phase of the aggression cycle they are in to implement appropriate intervention. 6. Individual cues, such as what the client is saying, changes in the client's voice—volume, pitch, speed; changes in the client's facial expression and behavior can help the nurse identify when aggressive behavior is coming up.	Assessment and effective interventions with angry or hostile clients can often prevent aggressive episodes. Early assessment, judicious use of medications, and verbal interaction with an angry client can often prevent anger from escalating into physical aggression. The data from the interview will help the nursing plan for nursing intervention to prevent harmful situations.
Be aware of factors that boost violent behavior and utilize verbal communication or PRN medication, restraint, and legal requirement.	Decide and act quickly. Warning signs of agitation include restlessness, verbal cues, motor activity pacing, speaking louder, verbal cues, threats, decreased frustration tolerance, and frowning or clenching fists. If the client is severely agitated, medication may be necessary to decrease the agitation.
Reduce external stimulation by turning the stereo or television off or lowering the volume, dropping the lights, and asking other clients, visitors, or others to leave the area.	The client is not capable of dealing with stimuli overload when agitated.
If the client communicates with you (verbally or nonverbally) that they feel hostile or destructive, try to help them express these feelings in non-destructive ways (e.g., use communication techniques or take the client to the gym for physical exercise).	The client can try performing positive behaviors with you in a nonthreatening environment and learn to focus on conveying emotions rather than acting out.
Serenely and deferentially assure the client that you will provide control if they cannot control themself, but do not threaten the client.	The client may fear the loss of control and be afraid of what they may do if they begin to express anger. Showing that you are in control without competing with the client can reassure them without lowering their self-esteem.
Encourage clients to state anger appropriately as a model and use roleplaying assertive communication techniques. Use "I" statements that speak of feelings and are specific to the situation, for example, "I feel angry when you interrupt me," or	The 'I' statements are a suitable expression of anger and can lead to creative problem-solving discussions and reduced anger.

Implementation (* Apply telenursing)	Rationale
"I am angry that you changed the work schedule without talking to me." *	
Enable weapon removal; try to kick it out of the client's hand.	Having a weapon increases your physical vulnerability.
The nurse needs to call outside assistance (especially if the client has a gun). When this is done, total accountability is delegated to the external authorities.	Exceeding the nurse's abilities may place you in grave danger. It is unnecessary to deal with a situation beyond your control or assume personal risk.
Report the in-charge nurse and supervisor in a (potentially) aggressive situation; convey to them your appraisal of the case and the requirement for help, the client's name, care plan, and orders for injection, seclusion, or restraint.	You may need support from staff members who are unfamiliar with this client. They will be able to help you more successfully and safely if they are aware of this information.
Follow the hospital staff guideline (e.g., use an intercom system to page "Code, [area]"); then, if needed, have one staff member meet the additional staff at the unit door to provide them with the client's name, situation, goal, plan, and so forth.	The need for help may be instant in a crisis. Any detail given to the arriving staff will ensure safety and helpfulness in dealing with this client.
Be aware of physical restraints or techniques with indication.	The client has a right to the least limits possible for safety and prevention of destructive behavior.
Remain aware of the client's body space or territory; do not trap the client.	Potentially violent people have a body space zone up to four times larger than that of other people. It would help if you stayed farther away from them for them not to feel trapped or threatened.
Talk with the client in a low, calm voice. Call the client by their name; tell the client your name and where you are.	Using a low voice may help prevent increasing agitation.
Tell the client what you will do and what you are doing. Use simple, straightforward, direct speech; repeat if necessary. Do not threaten the client, but state limits and expectations.	The client may be disoriented or unaware of what is happening.
When a decision has been made to subdue or restrain, the client acts quickly and cooperatively with other staff members. Tell the client that they will be controlled, suppressed, or secluded; allow 110 bargaining after the decision has been made. Reassure the client that they will not be hurt, and that restraint or seclusion is to ensure safety.	The client's ability to understand the situation and process information is impaired. Clear limits let the client know what is expected of them.
While subduing or restraining the client, talk with other staff members to ensure coordination of effort (e.g., do not attempt to carry the client until you are sure that everyone is ready).	Firm limits must be set and maintained. Bargaining interjects doubt and will undermine the limit.
Do not strike the client.	Direct verbal communication will promote cooperation and safety.
Do not help to restrain or subdue the client if you are angry (if enough other staff members are present).	The physical safety of the client is a priority.
Develop and practice consistent restraint techniques as part of nursing orientation and continue education.	Consistent techniques let each staff person know what is expected and will increase safety and effectiveness.

Implementation (* Apply telenursing)	Rationale
Develop instructions on safe techniques for carrying out with clients. Obtain additional staff assistance when needed. Have someone clear furniture and so forth from the area where you will be taking the client.	Consistent techniques increase safety and effectiveness. Transporting an agitated client can be unsafe if attempted without enough help and sufficient space.
When placing the client in restraint or seclusion, tell them what you are doing and why (e.g., to regain control or protect the client from injuring themself or others). Use simple, concise language in a non-judgmental manner.	The client's ability to understand what is happening to them may be impaired.
Give information to the client about where they are, that they will be safe, and the staff members that will take care of them. Tell the client how to summon the staff. Reorient the client or repeat to them the reason for restraint, as necessary.	Being placed in seclusion or restraint can be frightening for a client. Your assurance may aid in alleviating their fears.
Cautiously observe the client and promptly complete documentation regarding the hospital policy. Bear in mind the likely legal implications.	Correct, complete documentation is essential, as restraint, seclusion, assault, and so forth are events that may result in legal action.
Administer medication safely; prepare correct dosage, identify suitable sites for administration, withdraw plunger to aspirate for blood, and so forth.	When you are under stressful events and pressure to move fast, the risk of errors in dosage or administration of medication increases.
Keep away from needlestick injury and other injuries that may expose the client's blood/body fluids.	Hepatitis A or C, HIV, and other diseases are transmitted by blood or body fluids contact.
Monitor the client for medications' side effects and side effects and provide care as appropriate [14].	Medication treatment can have adverse effects, such as allergic reactions, hypotension, and pseudo-parkinsonian symptoms.
Talk with other clients after the situation is resolved; allow them to express feelings about the situation.*	The other clients have their own needs and problems. Be careful not to give attention only to the client acting out.

Table 6.
Implementation and rationale.

increased food consumption. It is known that psychological stress can alter both the quantity (there is usually an increased food intake) and quality (typically with high sugar or carbohydrate content) of food. Besides, stress-induced alterations in food intake can, in turn, influence mood 30,31. The literature has also demonstrated concern about food (often unhealthy) intake as a mechanism to cope with stress. It can be considered valid also in the context of this research. People who reported not "feeling sheltered at home" felt more psychological distress and poorer well-being. This is consistent with the evidence about the health benefits of cohabiting and the adverse effects of isolation (i.e., the state quarantine).

3.5 The barriers to telenursing during the pandemic

Implementing existing healthcare systems poses some potentially deterring and serious risks, such as confidentiality breaches, identity theft, technological breakdowns, and incompatibilities. Therefore, electronic records should not be hastily integrated into healthcare systems without proper precautions.

4. Conclusion

Telenursing, increasing diffusion and adoption of this type of work organization. The consequences of the COVID-19 pandemic and lockdown impact well-being and psychological distress experienced and are at risk of unhealthy eating behaviors and increased cigarette smoking or substance abuse, especially among those with higher education levels who live alone. Occupational physicians may play a central role in that process even through health promotion campaigns (healthy diets, tobacco smoking cessation) and supporting nurses in the risk assessment.

In order to provide nursing care to angry, hostile, or aggressive clients, nurses should identify the strategies to manage angry feelings, assessing assertive communication and conflict resolution. Enhancing these skills in dealing with behavioral problems in schizophrenic client will help nurses work more effectively with clients; the care of potentially aggressive clients should be discussed with experienced nurses, and nurses should be trained not to take the client's anger or aggressive behavior personally. Moreover, telenursing is a low-cost and free resource that will be the strategy for considering while providing care for the COVID-19 pandemic.

Conflict of interest

The authors declare no conflict of interest.

Author details

Ek-Uma Imkome
Faculty of Nursing, Thammasat University, Pratumtane, Thailand

*Address all correspondence to: ek-uma@nurse.tu.ac

References

[1] Rizk S, Bahia S. Effect of Tele-Nursing Education Program on Nurses' Compliance with Standard Precautions during COVID- 19 Pandemic. Assiut Scientific Nursing Journal. 2021;**9**(25): 10-19. DOI: 10.21608/asnj.2021. 73190.1166

[2] Raesi R, Shaye ZA, Saghari S. et al. The impact of education through nurse-led telephone follow-up (telenursing) on the quality of life of COVID-19 patients. Journal of the Egyptian Public Health Association. 2021;**96**:30. DOI: 10.1186/ s42506- 021-00093-y

[3] Bennett S, Agostinho S, Lockyer L. The process of designing for learning: Understanding university teachers' design work. Educational Technology Research and Development, 2017;**65**(1): 125-145. DOI: 10.1007/ s11423-016-9469-y

[4] Beebe DW, Fallone G, Godiwala N, Flanigan M, Martin D, Schaffner L, et al. Feasibility andbehavioral effects of an at-home multi-night sleeprestriction protocol for adolescents.Journal of ChildPsychology and Psychiatry. 2008; **49**:915-923

[5] Gidora H, Borycki EM, Kushniruk AW. Effects of telenursing triage and advice on healthcare costs and resource use. Studies in Health Technology and Informatics. 2019;**257**:133-139

[6] Jerant AF, Azari R, Martinez C, Nesbitt TS. A randomized trial of telenursing to reduce hospitalization for heart failure: Patient-centered outcomes and nursing indicators. Home Health Care Services Quarterly. 2003;**22**(1): 1-20. DOI: 10.1300/J027v22n01_01

[7] Imkome E, Yunibhund J, Chaiyawat W. A path analysis of psychotic symptoms among persons with schizophrenia using methamphetamines. Walailak Journal of Science and Technology. 2019;**16**(4): 283-294

[8] Allott K, Van-Der-El K, Bryce S, Hetrick S, Hamilton M, Killackey E, et al. Compensatory interventions for Cognitive impairments in psychosis: A systematic review and meta-analysis. Schizophrenia Bulletin. 2020;***46***(4): 869-883

[9] McGurk SR, Mueser KT, Pascaris A. Cognitive training and supported employment for persons with severe mental illness: One-year results from a randomized controlled trial. Schizophrenia Bulletin. 2005;**31**(4): 898-909

[10] Vauth R, Corrigan PW, Clauss M, Dietl M, Dreher-Rudolph M, Stieglitz R-D, et al. Cognitive strategies versus self-management skills as adjunct to vocational rehabilitation. Schizophrenia Bulletin. 2005;**31**(1):55-66

[11] Twamley EW, Vella L, Burton CZ, Heaton RK, Jeste DV. Compensatory cognitive training for psychosis: Effects in a randomized controlled trial. The Journal of Clinical Psychiatry. 2012; **73**(9):3529. DOI: 10.4088/JCP.12m07686

[12] Kirkpatrick B, Tek C. Schizophrenia: Clinical features and psychopathology concepts. Comprehensive textbook of psychiatry. 2005;**1**:1416-1436

[13] Imkome EU. Development and psychometric testing of the Thai impact and burden of care scale for caregivers of persons with schizophrenia and co-occurring methamphetamine use. F1000Research. 2021;**10**:484

[14] Imkome EU, Waraassawapati K. Perspectives and experiences of primary caregivers of individuals with Schizophrenia in Thailand. Issues in Mental Health Nursing. 2018;**39**(10): 858-864

[15] Keltner NL, Schwecke LH, Bostrorn CE. Psychiatric Nursing. 5th ed. St. Louis: Mosby, Inc; 2007

Chapter 4

Music as a Psychosocial Intervention with People Suffering from Schizophrenia: Challenges in Practice and Research

Inge Nygaard Pedersen, Lars Ole Bonde, Niels Jørgensen Hannibal, Charlotte Lindvang, Silvia Beatriz Jensen and Lars Rye Bertelsen

Abstract

In this chapter, we will present and reflect on challenges concerning clinical experiences and research within the area of music therapy as a psychosocial intervention for people suffering from schizophrenia. Two manuals for applying music therapy activities in two conditions in a research study were developed. The manual for the experimental group is based on intervention guidelines as a tool of engagement and regulation for the patient suffering from schizophrenia—simultaneously emphasizing an awareness of the position regarding closeness/distance and listening attitudes concerning the music therapist. Short descriptions of international research in the form of Cochrane- and meta-reviews will follow with an emphasis on presenting formulated needs in design developments for future studies. The description of a new Danish assessor- and patient-blinded randomized, controlled trial regarding music therapy vs. music listening for negative symptoms in schizophrenia will follow. We aimed at including these formulated needs of design development in the study, and in this chapter, we identify and describe different kinds of challenges emerging through our study, and we give some suggestions on how to cope with these. Finally, we discuss the complexity of doing controlled trials and using blinded research designs with this vulnerable population.

Keywords: music therapy, psychosocial intervention, schizophrenia, challenges in clinical practice, challenges in evidence-based research

1. Introduction

Music applied as a tool for rehabilitation and psychotherapy has grown very much during the last 50 years worldwide. Music therapy as a professional academic discipline is a training offered in almost every country around the world.

Music therapy can be performed in an active or a receptive form. In active music therapy, music improvisation can be used as a means of symbolically expressing emotions, sensations, and memories through which clients can gather personal insight and develop coping strategies. These same emotions, sensations, and memories can be evoked by guided music listening, thus hereby facilitating multi-modal imagery also potentially leading to personal insight. Often emotions are dealt with that human beings for some reason are not able to express through words. The use of music can further be a way of regulating arousal, reducing pain or alleviating insomnia, where music is applied as music medicine.

In this chapter, we will focus on music therapy as a means to reduce negative symptoms of schizophrenia such as social withdrawal, low motivation, and poor ability for contact and communication. The client population suffering from such negative symptoms is often chronically ill, and their quality of life is strongly reduced by the symptoms. Very few studies have investigated treatment possibilities for these symptoms, even if there is a correlation between negative symptoms and reduction in quality of key areas of life [1].

We will further focus on challenges for music therapists in clinical practice experienced through many years with this population and challenges in an evidence-based research study carried out in Denmark from 2016 to 2020. We will offer some reflections and solution ideas to these challenges and compare our study with similar previous studies presented in meta- and Cochrane reviews.

2. Challenges in clinical practice to be mirrored in a manual

2.1 Challenges in clinical practice

When offering music therapy to people suffering from schizophrenia with predominantly negative symptoms, it is not sufficient to be professional about applying music as a tool for symbolically expressing or evoking emotions, sensations, and memories. The music therapist also needs to be professional about obtaining contact or dialogs often at a very basic level. The music therapists must be extra aware of how they are present in the room—how they are listening, and which positions they take in the interplay, and most importantly, the timing of eventual shift in positions.

Danish music therapists have written about different stages in the treatment process, that the therapist needs to be aware of [2–4]. Examples can be: If the client accepts to participate in music therapy, it is often easy to motivate the client to play on an easily accessible music instrument such as a xylophone or a percussion instrument. But establishing a mutual interplay situation can be a big challenge. We have experienced clients who stop playing if they hear somebody else play at the same time or clients who are not able to listen to the music of someone else outside their own musical space. One possible intervention for the music therapist is to listen carefully and to reinforce the music of the client in a close imitation, so that the client does not even notice that he/she is imitated. This will provide no disturbances for the clients' musical space. Noticing this can be done meaningfully in musical interplay but would present quite meaningless in verbal interplay. Gradually, in such a first phase of starting interplay, the therapist can move from a position of imitation to a position of matching, from where the therapist can try out some enticing and calling musical techniques to try to be allowed to enter the musical world of the client. Most often the client allows short interruptions in his/her ongoing music expressions—often without starting or ending points or dynamical changes. These short interruptions can give the therapist an idea of how the client reacts to disturbances, but mostly the client quite quickly returns to the safe private music space, where no one is allowed to enter. Often the therapist has to give up on being allowed to enter the music of the client in the first phase of music therapy and needs to stay in a position of matching the client musically. In matching, you stay close to certain elements of the client's music such as dynamics and rhythm, but may apply other sound colors or instruments at the same time.

In a second phase of music therapy, the music therapist can be more holding than matching—this means that the therapist can support the music of the client in different ways such as grounding and framing and—leave the soloist position to the client. In this phase, it is not so much a question of being allowed to enter the music of the client—it is more about extending the expression of the client either with smooth music ornamentation or by supplying the music with a rhythmical or tonal center, from where the client can play further in his/her way. The interplay is still fully on the premises of the client, but the client allows music accompaniment to take place. It can provide a resonance of feeling all alone by the therapist, which again can be a counter-transference feeling toward the client's transference [5–7].

In a third phase of the music therapy—with the right timing (when the client is ready), the therapist can consciously try to disturb the music of the client, take a more contrasting role, and encourage and provoke the client to react to these contrasts. This phase often provides breakthrough experiences for the client, who often reacts quite dynamically as if being drawn out of a safe bubble where well-known patterns are left behind. A real interplay can occur in the here and now. It might be only for less than a minute, and the client may regret it afterward and ask for such experiences not to be repeated. It is audible though in the musical interplay in a fourth phase, that the client is more present in the music—more listening to others and there is a more equal, playful and independent interplay in the therapist/client dyad although the music can still float together.

2.2 Creating a manual mirroring clinical challenge

In creating a manual for a research study for this population, clinical experiences as presented above and many other experiences need to be mirrored in the structure of the manual. We were inspired by [8], who suggest guiding principles rather than factual descriptions in a manual for complex interventions. We were also inspired by [9], who recommend a four-level structure, which has already been applied by other music therapists such as [10–12].

The four levels consist of the following: (1) Unique and Essential Therapeutic Principles (principles that are central and defining), (2) Essential but not Unique Therapeutic Principles (principles that are also essential to other methods), (3) Acceptable but not Necessary Therapeutic Principles (principles that are not essential or defining to a certain approach in music therapy), and finally (4) Not Acceptable—Proscribed Therapeutic Principles (principles that are strongly contradictory to this approach).

2.2.1 The manual for the experimental group

For our study, we reflected that the manual for the experimental group (group I), performed by an educated music therapist unknown to the participant, should be flexible for clinical practice and there should be a possibility of multiple choices of music therapy techniques tailored to the need of the single client. Thus, the principles were mostly guiding toward a certain awareness of distance and closeness in the presence of the therapist and awareness of the different needs of the client in different phases of the therapy process. Moreover, in the manual, the therapist is guided to not push the client and at the same time being sensitive to activation possibilities. Further, guiding principles concerned building alliance at a safe tempo for the participant, keeping stable frames and awareness of being both inviting for sharing problems, and simultaneously being supportive toward resources emerging in the therapeutic relationship. Following are examples of the therapeutic principles at level 1 and 4:

1) Unique and Essential Principles

- Switching between closeness and distance in the therapist/client relationship in an awareness of the right timing.

- Considering the negative symptoms as something "between us." This between us can in the right timing be due to mutual investigation—being investigative, resonant, and aware what the symptoms are eventually expressing.

and

4) Not Acceptable—Proscribed Principles sound:

- Being guided solely by methodological or theoretical perspectives without involving the perspective of the client and the current relationship.

- Being judgmental or dismissive of the participant's experience of the world.

2.2.2 The manual for the control group

For the control group (group II), our rationale for the music listening condition was that we wanted an active offer of intervention for both groups. We did not want the study to examine music therapy added to treatment as usual versus treatment as usual alone as has been mostly applied in research sources involving this population. Moreover, for ethical reasons, we did not want half of the clients to face challenging screening procedures without being offered an intervention. We decided to offer group II music listening to playlists developed by music therapists, where the intervention is performed by a caregiver unknown to the participant. The caregivers, performing group II intervention, were instructed by music therapists on how to apply the playlists in an App called *The Music-Star* [13]. The caregivers trained for this intervention all needed previous experiences in working or being with the population under investigation. We also wanted a condition for group II including music as our study was blinded for participants and screening nurses. Thus, one of the possible activities in the music therapy group I became the only possible music activity in group II. This condition created a situation where we could name both conditions as music therapy activities—and inform the participants that we were examining two different music therapy interventions.

All performers of interventions in group I and group II were called therapists, and all interventions took place in the same locations equipped for music therapy and with a firm weekly meeting time. We also formulated that the therapist performing group II should not be allowed to actively build a therapeutic alliance and should not enter a therapeutic dialog. The therapist should solely listen to the client without verbal interventions.

For this group II condition, we did not apply all four therapeutic principles in the same form as for the group I condition. We simply applied three short principles:

(1) You must, (2) You can, (3) You are not allowed to, as presented in the following examples from level 1 and level 3:

1) You must:

- 1. Be motivating and firm around listening to music from the playlists (The Music-Star App). Music listening should preferably take place in each session.

- Apply "prepared ready answers" if asked about your profession/role (from the list of ready answers).

3) You are not allowed to:

- Actively ask about the participant's current life situation or life story. If the participant takes an initiative to share life events, do listen in an engaged manner, but do not offer to clarify or confront comments or answers.

- Perform music actively (sing or play) alone or together with the participant.

- Talk with the participant about how she/he is influenced by or experiences the music.

Thus, we could be rather flexible with the two intervention conditions and give some space for the therapist to meet the need of the participants in different ways. Simultaneously, we needed to be rigor with our research design as this is demanded in the Danish health system, but it is also asked for in meta-reviews of previous research studies with this population.

3. Challenges in developing a research design as mirrored in the results

3.1 Challenges in developing a research design

In 2015, when we planned to establish a research study in Denmark examining the possibility of reducing negative symptoms of people suffering from schizophrenia through music therapy, we were inspired by recommendations presented in previous Cochrane reviews such as [14, 15]. During our study, similar and further recommendations were emphasized in several meta-reviews that supported our choices concerning a rigorous design among others [16–19]. The recommendations included: (1) applying a more rigorous research design than had been the case in previous studies, (2) applying an active control condition, not solely measuring music therapy added to treatment as usual versus treatment as usual alone, (3) distinguishing between primary and secondary negative symptoms, (4) clarifying the music therapy condition and who would be performing the intervention.

Therefore, we developed a randomized, controlled, assessor- and patient-blinded trial, which was carried out from 2016 to 2020, after having developed the protocol design during 2015. Based on power calculation, we aimed at a minimum of 90 and a maximum of 120 participants. This study was a collaboration between music therapy researchers from Aalborg University and psychiatrists from Aalborg University Hospital, Psychiatry. Our aim of the study is clarified in the following citation:

"The ambition in the present study was to apply a rigorous research design with manualized interventions, standardized outcomes and an active control condition, in order to reduce the risk of observing Hawthorne effects when studying adjunct music therapy. We further established a blinded condition and ensured that all potential participants received the same information ..." [20] p. 6.

We decided to develop our research design as similar as possible to a medical study design, well aware that this was an ambitious task with this vulnerable population.

As already mentioned, we created a control condition including music, and we even ensured blinding for the participants and the assessors (project nurses). The blinding seemed to be successful, as only three participants from group II expressed that they did not get real music therapy, and they all dropped out during treatment. The design included a big number of measurement tools, which showed to be challenging for the participants.

3.1.1 Measurement tools

We applied two standardized tools for measuring symptoms of schizophrenia—both negative and positive, namely the Positive and Negative Syndrome Scale (PANSS) [21], where we focused on four items of the negative subscale: Blunded affect N1; Emotional withdrawal N2; Poor rapport N3; Passive/apathetic social withdrawal N4; The subscale had to show 4 or >4 on two of those parameters for the participant to be included.

The positive subscale 1–7 had to show no higher than 28 in total for the participant to be included in the study. We also applied the Brief Negative Symptom Scale (BNSS) [22] to have a broader sense of the symptoms. We included two further scales to ensure that primary negative symptoms—not secondary negative symptoms such as depression or side effects from medication—were present, namely the Calgary Depression Scale [23] for Schizophrenia (CDSS) and the UKU scale [24] measuring general effects of side effects induced by treatment with antipsychotics. UKU is an acronym for the Danish name "Udvalg for Kliniske Undersøgelser" (Task Force for Clinical Investigations).

Other measurement tools applied were the Global Assessment of Functioning (GAF), WHOQOL-Bref (Quality of Life), and Helping Alliance Questionnaire, patient version (Haq-II).

The high number of measurement tools provided that every screening procedure lasted a minimum of 1.5 hours. The participants were screened before inclusion, after 15 sessions and after 25 sessions. The Helping Alliance Questionnaire was applied also after session 5 but not before inclusion.

For further information on the different measurement tools, see [25].

3.1.2 Other inclusion and exclusion criteria

The participants included were aged 18–65, and they had to have a diagnosis of schizophrenia stated (ICD-10, F20) more than 2 years ago. To be included they could not have had a change in medicine within the last month or have been hospitalized within the last 3 months. A significant drug dependency, conflicting with participation in the study, could also lead to exclusion. Finally, potential participants were not allowed to have received individual music therapy within the last 2 months. This last criterion was based on a direct translation of a criterion from medical studies. Normally it takes 2 months to eliminate the effect of medicine, and this effect needs to be eliminated to ensure that the new trial is not influenced by previous medicine (here in the form of individual music therapy).

When participants were included in the study and randomized to one of two intervention arms, they could be excluded if they were absent from more than five of the 25 sessions or if more than 30 days passed between two sessions. They could also be excluded if a significant shift in medicine was needed during the trial or if they were hospitalized for more than 3–4 days. In all cases when a participant did not turn up for a session and had not canceled before the session, the therapist phoned the participant to ensure that they were OK with the choice of not attending the session. All therapists actively gave notice to the participants, if they had been absent for four or five sessions, that they should be aware that another absence would result in exclusion from the study.

Twenty-five sessions of interventions in both groups were chosen based on previous research [26], that the dose-response effect of music therapy in work with clients with low motivation and complex symptoms is higher between 16 and 51 sessions and not so high between 3 and 10 sessions. We made a power calculation based on previous studies, stating a higher number than in several previous studies due to having a control group in this study. The calculation suggested min. 90 and max. 120 participants.

3.2 Challenges in recruitment processes

We planned a recruitment process stating that the researchers—primarily the principal investigator and the research coordinator—planned and performed several initial information meetings with institutions and institution units, where potential participants were living or a place they were visiting daily. As we searched for participants being diagnosed more than 2 years ago, we recruited solely outpatients at hospitals or social institutions. We planned to identify one contact person among the staff at each institution/unit, and we intended to instruct this person comprehensively on how to inform and encourage potential participants. The research coordinator would keep a weekly telephone contact with all informants, but we soon realized that this procedure did not work.

Two challenges emerged during the recruitment phase: Firstly, it happened that the informants forgot to inform other team members or potential participants, or -if they informed other team members, these team members forgot the message as soon as they left the room. The team members of these institutions told us that they simply were overloaded with working issues and not always able to perform this new task, even if they were motivated to. Secondly, team members often had a protective attitude toward their clients. So, if they thought that a potential participant was not able to join 25 sessions of music therapy activities, they did not inform the client. We tried to solve these challenges by simply performing many more meetings at each institution and by being allowed to be connected directly with potential participants, and to answer all their questions and comment on their doubts. For some periods in the recruitment phase, the research task grew from a part-time job to a full-time job for the coordinator and the principal investigator—an extra expense not originally included in the research budget.

A third challenge in the recruitment process was the fact that we were not allowed to contact any staff member at any institution until a collaboration contract was signed by the head of a mental health center, often including many institutions. This procedure was very time-consuming, and more center managers did not want to sign such a contract, which meant that even if we aimed at performing a national study among all five regions in Denmark, we were not able to recruit in two out of five regions. One region was not a possibility as no music therapists were working in mental health institutions in this region at the time of the project. In the end, only two regions signed a contract. In some regions, the healthcare institutions were overloaded by problems from just having a new electronic online journaling practice installed, which caused heavy problems for the daily work of all healthcare professionals, and we unfortunately started our study at the same time. As we were not able to counter these challenges, we limited our study to two regions, which again gave us fewer chances to obtain our estimated number of participants.

A fourth challenge was an unforeseen quick shift of staff members working in mental health, which took place at several institutions in Denmark in the years of the study. For this study, it meant that instead of one psychiatrist researcher, three psychiatrist researchers became involved in the study during the years. We were only allowed to recruit when a psychiatrist researcher was involved, so these transitions from one psychiatrist researcher to the next created longer phases during the study, where we were not able to recruit. It was an important lesson to witness how influential structural elements as described above can influence the recruitment process and prolong the study.

3.2.1 Challenges in the inclusion screening procedure

When a potential participant showed interest in the study, the local contact person would reach out to the research coordinator. The coordinator aimed at collecting at least three participants or more to arrange a screening meeting with our two project nurses—mostly at the institution of the participants so it could take place at a familiar place for the potential participants. These screening procedures thus involved traveling and sometimes staying overnight for the project nurses. We, therefore, decided to deviate from the original plan that the same two project nurses should do all screening procedures to ensure screening compliance and trained and included more project nurses living in another Region. The two original project nurses further trained five accessors during the study period.

A total of 199 participants showed interest in the study for whom a screening procedure was planned. A huge challenge emerged already here, where 62 of those clients either did not turn up or withdrew their consent during the screening procedure. Participants were offered a taxi for traveling to and from the procedure, and we planned the procedure to take place close to where potential participants were living. Before the start of the screening procedure, they were informed by the project nurse about the project and the screening procedure and—among others about the fact that a video recording of 20 minutes was part of the screening procedure to ensure screening validity. Especially this part of the screening procedure caused problems for several potential participants. Further, they had to sign an informed consent form "to provide allowance to receive information of diagnosis, medical information, and hospitalization history of the single participant. If this is not possible, the client cannot be included in the study." [25]. So many factors could provide that the potential participant became insecure or regretted just before or during the planned screening procedure.

Seventy-seven potential participants were not included even if they went through the screening procedure. We can identify some factors causing this challenge. Firstly, in the beginning, mostly clients with an interest in music were referred as their contact person interpreted that this had to be a condition. This happened even if we emphasized very clear at all information meetings that we were searching for participants with negative symptoms and that they did not need to have an interest in music. Secondly, many participants wanted to give the screening project nurse a positive picture of their abilities. As an example, if they were registered for activities that they never attended, they answered questions about these activities as if they were joining them and thus did not meet the criteria of the sum of negative symptoms.

The first challenge listed here was resolved when the researchers themselves gradually were allowed to have the direct information task with the potential participants. The second challenge we solved by the screening nurse starting to tell the potential participant before the start of the screening that the screening was not about giving a positive but a realistic picture of oneself. We lost a further three included participants before randomization, because one was moving to another town in Denmark, and two participants withdrew their consent after inclusion but before randomization. Thus, we ended up with 57 included participants.

For each participant being included and randomized to one of two interventions, the coordinator had to connect the participant with one of our 13 therapists at a location as close as possible to the living place of the participant. All together 10 locations were equipped for music therapy activities. If more than 2 weeks passed from the screening date to the first intervention date, the participant had to go through a new screening procedure. This criterion illustrates how quickly symptoms can change within this population, and that each screening procedure is a picture of the here and now situation for the participant.

The coordinator collected session schedules filled in by each therapist and organized all screening procedures ensuring they were performed after 15 and after 25 sessions. The Haq-II questionnaire was filled out after 5, 15, and 25 sessions, performed by either the research coordinator or the principal investigator. The principal investigator performed all semistructured interviews after 1 month follow-up.

3.3 Challenges in design and recruitment as mirrored in the results

In total, 57 participants were randomized (28 in group I and 29 in group II). We did not meet the aim of power calculation. Of these participants, 39 completed the first 15 sessions (25 in group I and 14 in group II) and 29 completed all 25 sessions (17 in group I and 12 in group II).

The Demographics of study participants did not show differences in duration of illness, age at inclusion, PANSS negative subscale, sex, substance misuse, schizophrenia subtype, and education (**Table 1**).

At baseline we observed no difference between groups in any of the measurement tools (PANSS total score, PANSS subscale scores, BNSS total score, BNSS subscale scores, CDSS, GAF, WHO-QoL total score, and Haq II total score) (**Table 2**).

PANSS, positive and negative symptom scale; BNSS, brief negative symptom scale; GAF, global assessment of functioning; WHO-QoL, World Health Organization quality of life; HAQ II, Helping Alliance Questionnaire (Patient version II); CI, confidence interval.

Our primary outcome was stated as the results of the PANSS negative subscales—total scale, and as a result, we found no significant differences between the two groups. Surprisingly both intervention groups showed a significant reduction in negative symptoms from baseline to 25 weeks of treatment.

Both **Figures 1** and **2** were first edited by Frontiers in Psychiatry. Clinical Trial, published 21. December 2021. doi: 10.3389/fpsyt.2021.738810. Unfortunately, an error in the data recording has been detected since this publication, changing the number of Music Listening, 25 weeks to 12 instead of previously 13 in both figures. This error does not influence the result.

	Music therapy (n = 28)	Music listening (n = 29)	p-value
Sex[a]			
Male	18 (66.7%)	16 (57.1%)	0.6
Age at baseline[b]	40.7 (13.2)	36.5 (11.3)	0.2
Duration of illness[b]	9.0 (7.9)	7.0 (8.7)	0.5
Education[a]			0.3
Law-mandated school	7 (25.0%)	6 (20.7%)	
Grammar school (gymnasium or similar)	8 (28.6%)	10 (34.5%)	
Short vocation-oriented courses	5 (17.9%)	2 (6.9%)	
Vocational/apprenticeship training	4 (14.3%)	8 (27.6%)	
University training	1 (3.6%)	3 (10.3%)	
Other	1 (3.6%)	—	
Schizophrenia subtype[a,c]			0.6
Paranoid Schizophrenia	17 (73.9%)	19 (70.4%)	
Hebephrenic schizophrenia	1 (4.3%)	—	
Undifferentiated schizophrenia	3 (13.0%)	5 (18.5%)	
Simple schizophrenia	1 (4.3%)	—	
Remaining subtypes	1 (4.3)	3 (11.1%)	
Misuse of alcohol or substances[a]	1 (3.6%)	1 (3.4%)	> 0.9

[a]*Frequency (%); p-value from Fisher's exact test.*
[b]*Mean (SD); p-value from two-sided t-test.*
[c]*Schizophrenia subtype data were missing for seven participants.*

Table 1.
Demographics of study participants.

	Intervention I		Intervention II	
	Mean	95% CI	Mean	95% CI
PANSS total	73.9	(69.0–78.8)	68.6	(65.1–72.1)
PANSS negative subscale	23.4	(21.7–25.1)	23.4	(21.4–25.4)
PANSS positive subscale	15.6	(13.6–17.7)	13.7	(12.3–15.1)
PANSS general subscale	34.9	(31.8–38.0)	31.5	(29.2–33.8)
BNSS total	37.4	(33.9–41.0)	36.2	(32.4–40.0)
BNSS anhedonia subscale	10.4	(9.4–11.4)	10.2	(9.0–11.4)
BNSS distress subscale	2.4	(1.8–2.9)	1.6	(0.9–2.2)
BNSS asociality subscale	5.5	(4.6–6.3)	5.2	(4.5–5.9)
BNSS avolition subscale	6.5	(5.8–7.1)	6.5	(5.7–7.2)
BNSS blunted affect subscale	7.9	(6.6–9.1)	7.9	(6.4–9.5)
BNSS alogia subscale	4.9	(3.8–6.1)	4.9	(3.9–5.8)
Calgary depression scale for schizophrenia	3.2	(2.1–4.3)	3.7	(2.9–4.4)
GAF	39.4	(36.4–42.3)	41.3	(38.7–43.8)
WHO-QoL total score	77.0	(71.8–82.1)	76.8	(71.8–81.8)

	Intervention I		Intervention II	
	Mean	**95% CI**	**Mean**	**95% CI**
WHO-QoL physical health domain raw score	20.8	(18.8–22.7)	21.9	(19.9–23.9)
WHO-QoL psychological domain raw score	15.6	(13.9–17.4)	14.3	(12.6–15.9)
WHO-QoL social relationships domain raw score	9.0	(8.4–9.7)	9.4	(8.5–10.3)
WHO-QoL environment domain raw score	24.9	(22.9–26.8)	26.0	(24.6–27.3)
HAQ II Helping Alliance Questionnaire	5.0	(4.6–5.3)	4.7	(4.4–5.1)

Table 2.
Baseline scores of study participants.

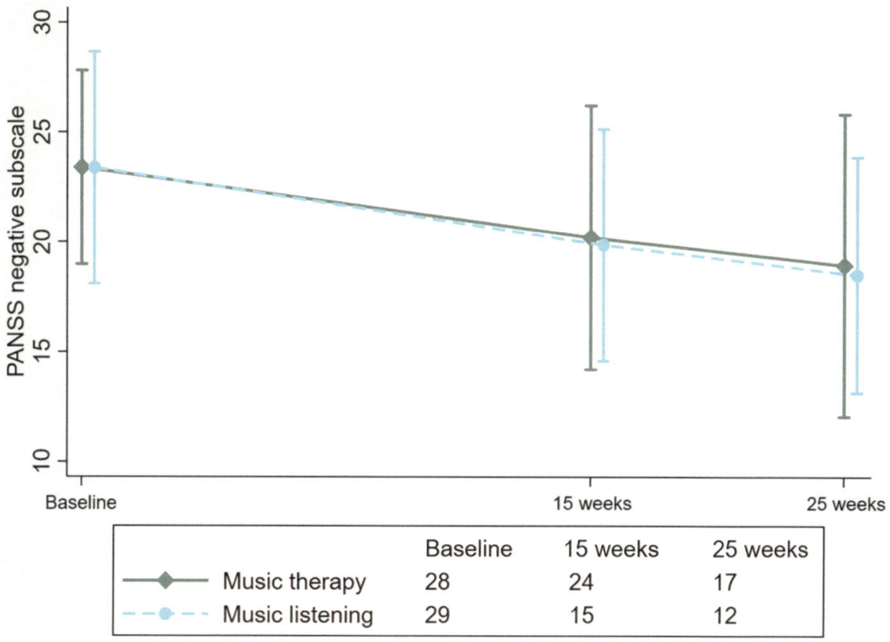

Figure 1.
Changes in positive and negative syndrome scale (PANSS), negative subscale in the intention to treat population.

A qualitative analysis of the semistructured interviews, performed after 1 month after termination of 25 sessions, is under elaboration. We will bring a few citations from those interviews at the end of this chapter. We think the challenges addressed in this chapter are all elements providing the high dropout rate we had to face in the study.

3.3.1 Discussion on challenges mirrored in the results

After completing this study, the question is how we can understand the results in the light of the challenges of the study?

First, we were aware that applying a study design, as close to a medical design as possible for this vulnerable population, is bound to cause challenges. We were prepared for this but not for such big scale challenges. We were prepared that some

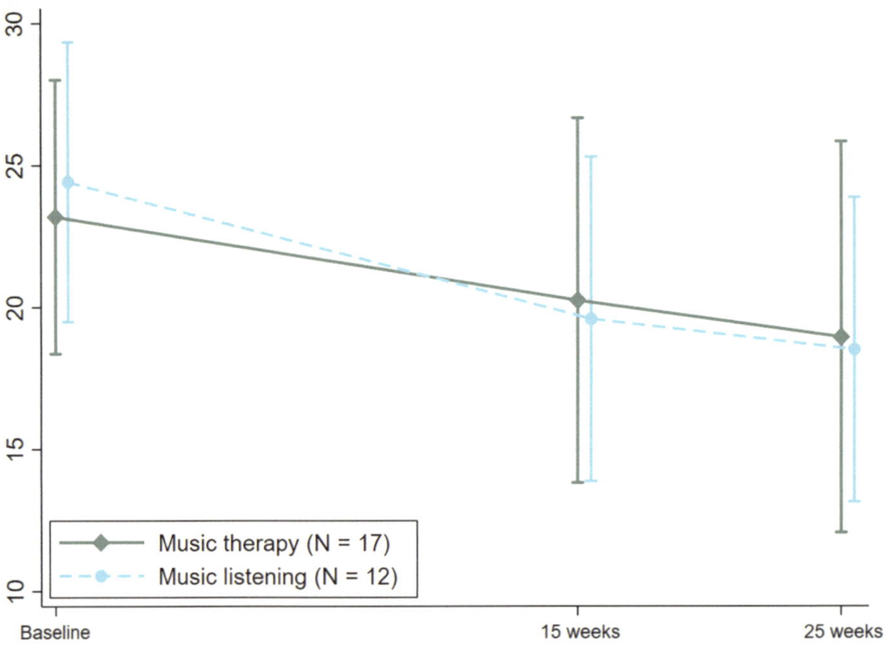

Figure 2.
Changes in positive and negative syndrome scale (PANSS), negative subscale in the completer's population.

potential participants would either not show interest or might regret just before the initial screening procedure; but we were not prepared for such a high number of screening failures. This fact can reflect that the protecting attitude of some staff members seems realistic. On the other hand, we also had participants completing screening, where the team members told us, that they did not think the participant could turn up for any session, but the participant eventually completed all 25 sessions. Retrospectively, the results may reflect that the screening procedures were too comprehensive, and that too many measurement tools caused challenges, and further, that 25 sessions may have been a bit scary to face before start for some potential participants. Simultaneously, we initially agreed that we wanted to meet the demands for more rigorous designs. Seen in the light of the estimated power calculation, we recruited very few; but seen in the light of the design applied, we have had reactions from professionals working with this population who were surprised that we were able to include 57 participants.

The outcomes of the study in our opinion mirror that this population does change rather quickly in mood and in showing courage, and they seem to easily be comprehensively influenced by these changes.

Research shows that negative symptoms provide problems in treating people suffering from schizophrenia, as psychopharmaceuticals and other treatment are only effectual to a lesser extent for this patient population [1, 27]. From this perspective, we think it is positive that the study shows a significant reduction of negative symptoms for both groups.

An important finding was that both interventions showed improvement in the level of negative symptoms for the participants, who were able to participate in the final assessment after 25 sessions. The data do not reveal what parameters predict the profile of the participants, who would profit from each of the two interventions. The underpower of the study is also important in this respect, as a larger number might have changed the between group outcomes. Some clients benefitted more from music therapy, where several techniques were applied, and the therapist aimed to tailor the process of the case to the needs of the client. This is a more active intervention, where the relationship between the therapist and the client is an important part of the treatment process. Other clients benefitted more from being in a location with a carefully listening person, with no demands of being active other than choosing some music from the playlist to listen to. This intervention form can be seen more like a music activity, where the building of alliance is less important in the treatment process.

In the interviews, more participants joining group II expressed that it was important for them just to turn up and to listen to some supportive music—not being asked about anything. As there was a bigger number of dropouts in group II than in group I from session 1 to session 15 (4 in group I and 13 in group II), it seems possible that intervention II could not engage the participant at the same level as intervention I. Only participants who wanted no engagement (no disturbance), but who benefitted from just getting out of their home once a week, seemed to continue the treatment in group II. These reflections need further research studies, and we can just learn from the fact that the mood and motivation are changing quickly for some participants in the population under investigation, and that these changes seem to have a comprehensive influence on the mental state of the participants. We acknowledge the benefit of giving patients, who are chronically ill, a chance to get out of their homes and feel good about it.

The music playlists selected for group II—a special compilation of playlists, also available as one possible intervention for group I—are specifically chosen by two music therapy researchers, who, from certain parameters on the intensity of the music, divided playlists into three different categories: (1) supportive music, (2) supportive and challenging music, and (3) challenging music [28]. In the present study, only music from the supportive category was included in the app.

In Denmark, it has been a practice for some years that music therapists employed in mental health hospital institutions do instruct other staff members on how to apply the playlists on the app called "The Music-Star" [13]. These playlists are applied for several other tasks, e.g., to try to avoid coercion and belt fixation, or the playlists are applied for helping clients with insomnia or restlessness e.g. Ref. [29]. In this respect, the results just confirm that both practices, which are already present in some mental health institutions, having music therapists employed, can be beneficial for people suffering from schizophrenia with predominantly negative symptoms. Both interventions call for a music therapist as part of the team.

This study has given much indispensable knowledge and experience for us as music therapy researchers. We hope to be able to apply this knowledge in future research designs, in qualitative or mixed-method research designs in the mental health system. We also hope that these research methods will achieve the same recognition as quantitative evidence-based research concerning treatment possibilities. We hope that these methods—at least for complex diagnoses and symptoms—can be as beneficial for informing the health system, about which treatment possibilities should be recommended as standard care. Thus, not only treatment manuals, but also research study designs could be tailored more toward the realistic possibilities of the potential participants. We have learned from this study that the many measurement tools and long screening procedures cause anxiety, insecurity, and dropout on a big scale. We recommend that future research in the field examines if other ways of gaining data could cause less dropout and still provide valid results.

As a final part of this paper, we want to give the word to the participants in the study. Without their contribution, none of these experiences would have been possible. These few citations are formulated by the participants during the semistructured interviews and translated by the authors:

- "I think it has reduced negative thoughts. It is helpful to just listen to music. I never thought of this before".

- "It is a really good treatment offer. It basically helped me to cope with life. It did not permanently remove the symptoms. During treatment the weeks were much better – it went down again towards the next session and after the session, it went up again. It needs to be a permanent offer – this will make the process more fluently – then it can be adjusted along the road".

- "I never thought that sitting and playing some piano keys could have any influence on one's mood. It had a huge effect. I have been happy on the days when I could go for a session and be in a very good mood the rest of such a day – even during a winter depression. Normally months pass between such happy mood days, and suddenly I had a weekly happy mood day. I never expected I could join 25 weeks' sessions – but I did!!!! Music can carry me out of the depressive part of me. This is necessary to act in life. The change in my state of being is slow, but it does move forward".

4. Conclusion

To conclude, clients diagnosed with schizophrenia and suffering from predominantly negative symptoms—also in social psychiatry—can benefit from either music therapy or music listening to special selected music play lists—here through the App *Music-Star*.

As explained in the text, most participants dropped out before, during or just after the first screening procedure. More participants dropped out between baseline and 15 sessions in intervention II than in intervention I, which could indicate that intervention I can motivate more clients to stay in the treatment situation. Still, we anticipate that many more patients can benefit from both interventions, when not being demanded to go through long screening processes, and when music therapy is integrated in the institution. It seems to be a future assessment task for music therapists to distinguish, which clients within this population can benefit most from which of the two intervention offers described here.

Acknowledgements

We would first of all like to say thank you to all the participants, who made this study possible. And all the members of the research team including psychiatrists, project nurses, therapists, statisticians, and other researchers in the steering group. We are grateful to Aalborg University and Aalborg University Hospital, Psychiatry, who supported this project throughout the many years. Finally, we want to thank the TRYG Foundation without whom we could never have performed this study. They gave us 400.000 euros to perform the study. Also, we want to thank the Obel Family Foundation, which provided money to equip some of the music therapy locations.

Conflict of interest

Lars Rye Bertelsen is coowner of the design rights for the Music-Star App. This app was developed in 2015–2016 in a joint venture between Aalborg University Hospital, Psychiatry, the private vendor AudioCura, ApS., and music therapists Helle Nystrup Lund and Lars Rye Bertelsen, who are both coowners of the design rights to the app. The remaining authors declare that the research was conducted in the absence of any commercial or financial relationships that could be construed as a conflict of interest.

Author details

Inge Nygaard Pedersen[1*], Lars Ole Bonde[2], Niels Jørgensen Hannibal[1], Charlotte Lindvang[1], Silvia Beatriz Jensen[3] and Lars Rye Bertelsen[4]

1 Aalborg University, Aalborg, Denmark

2 CREMAH, The Norwegian Academy of Music, Oslo, Norway

3 Private Practice, Aalborg, Denmark

4 Aalborg University Hospital, Aalborg, Denmark

*Address all correspondence to: inp@ikp.aau.dk

References

[1] SRT V, Schulte PF, de Hahn L. Treatment for negative symptoms in schizophrenia: A comprehensive review. Drugs. 2017;**77**:1423-1459

[2] Jensen B. Musikterapi med skizofrene – refleksioner ud fra en case. (Music therapy with people suffering from schizophrenia – Reflections based on a case). Musikterapi i Psykiatrien. Årsskrift 2, (Music Therapy in Mental Health. Vol.2). 2002;**2**:31-48. Available from: https://journals.aau.dk//index.php/MIPO

[3] Lindvang, C: Musikterapeutens rolle i opbygning af psykoterapeutisk relation med skizofrene. (The role of the music therapist in building a psychotherapeutic alliance with people suffering from schizophrenia). Musikterapi i Psykiatrien. Årsskrift 1. (Music Therapy in Mental Health. Vol. 1) 1998;1:45-64. Available from: https://journals.aau.dk//index.php/MIPOhttps://journals.aau.dk//index.php/MIPO

[4] Pedersen, IN: Music therapy as holding and re-organizing work with schizophrenic and psychotic patients. In: Wigram T, De Backer J, editors. Clinical Applications of Music Therapy in Psychiatry. London: Jessica Kingsley Publishers; 1999. pp. 24-44

[5] Pedersen IN. Counter transference in music therapy. A Phenomenological study on counter transference used as a clinical concept by music therapists working with musical improvisation in adult psychiatry [Dissertation]. Aalborg University; 2007. Available from: https://www.mt-phd.aau.dk/phd-theses/

[6] Pedersen IN. Musikterapeutens disciplinerede subjektivitet. (The disciplined subjectivity of the music therapist). Music and Psychology. Psyke & Logos. 2007;**28**(1):358-384

[7] Pedersen IN. En fænomenologisk undersøgelse af modoverføring i musikalsk improvisation i voksenpsykiatrien. En praksisbaseret og praksisrelateret forskningsundersøgelse. (A phenomenological examination of counter transference in musical improvisation in adult psychiatry. A practice based and practice related research study). Musikterapi I Psykiatrien. Årgang 5 (Music therapy in mental health. Vol. 5). 2008;**5**:30-46. Available from: https://journals.aau.dk//index.php/MIPO

[8] Hawe P, Shiell A, Riley T. Complex interventions: How "out of control" can a randomised controlled trial be? BMJ. 2004;**328**(7455):1561-1563

[9] Waltz J, Addis ME, Koerner K, Jacobson NS. Testing the integrity of a psychotherapy protocol: Assessment of adherence and competence. Journal of Consulting and Clinical Psychology. 1993;**61**(4):620-630

[10] Rolvsjord R, Gold C, Stige B. Research rigour and therapeutic flexibility: Rationale for a therapy manual developed for a randomized controlled trial. Nordic Journal of Music Therapy. 2005;**14**(14):15-32. DOI: 10.1080/08098130509478122

[11] Hannibal NJ, Pedersen IN, Bertelsen LR, Dammeyer C, Lund HN. Manual for procesorienteret musikterapi for personer med BPD. (A manual for process-based music therapy for persons suffering from BPD). Musikterapi i Psykiatrien Online (MIPO). 2012;7(2):64-80. DOI: 10.5278/ojs/mipo/401ctlm2

[12] Geretsegger M, Holck U, Bieleninik L, Gold C. Feasibility of a

trial on improvisational music therapy for children with autism spectrum disorder. Journal of Music Therapy. 2016;**53**(2):93-120

[13] Lund HN, Bertelsen LR, Bonde LO. Sound and music interventions in psychiatry at Aalborg university hospital. SoundEffects. 2016;**6**:48-68. DOI: 10.7146/se.v6i1.24912 26

[14] Gold C, TO H, Dahle T, Wigram T. Music therapy for schizophrenia or schizophrenia-like illnesses. Cochrane Data Base Systematic Reviews. 2005;**18**(2):CD0040025

[15] Mössler K, Chen X, TO H, Gold C. Music Therapy for People with Schizophrenia and Schizophrenia-like Disorders. The Cochrane Collaboration. Hoboken, NJ, USA: John Wiley & Sons Ltd.; 2011. DOI:1002/14651858. CD004025

[16] Lutgens D, Gariepy G, Malla A. Psychological and psychosocial interventions for negative symptoms in psychosis: Systematic review and meta-analysis. The British Journal of Psychiatry. 2017;**210**:324-332. DOI: 10.1192/bjp.bp.116.197103

[17] Tseng PT, Chen YW, Lin PY, Tu KY, Wang HY, Cheng YS, et al. Significant treatment effect of adjunct music therapy to standard treatment on the positive, negative, and mood symptoms of schizophrenic patients: A meta-analysis. BMC Psychiatry. 2016;**16**:16. DOI: 10.1186/s12888-016-0718-8

[18] Geretsegger M, Mossler KA, Bieleninik L, Chen XJ, Heldal TO, Gold C. Music therapy for people with schizophrenia and schizophrenia-like disorders. Cochrane Database of Systematic Reviews. 2017;**5**:CD004025. DOI: 10.1002/14651858.CD004025.pub4

[19] Jia R, Dandan L, Jingfen Y, Guangl L, Zihu W, Zhen W, et al. The effectiveness of adjunct music therapy for patients with schizophrenia: A meta-analysis. Psychiatry Research. 2020;**293**:3464. DOI: 10.1016/j.psychres.2020.113464

[20] Pedersen IN, Bonde LO, Hannibal Nielsen J, Aagaard J, Gold C, Bertelsen LR, et al. Music therapy vs. music listening for negative symptoms in schizophrenia: Randomized, controlled, assessor- and patient-blinded trial. Frontiers in Psychiatry. 2021;**12**:738810. DOI: 10.3389/fpsyt.2021.738810

[21] Kay SR, Fiszbein A, Opler LA. The positive and negative syndrome scale (PANSS) for schizophrenia. Schizophrenia Bulletin. 1987;**13**:261-276. DOI: 10.1093/schbul/13.2.261

[22] Kirkpatrick B, Strauss GP, Nguyen L, Fischer BA, Daniel DG, Cienfuegos A, et al. The brief negative symptom scale; psychometric properties. Schizophrenia Bulletin. 2011;**37**:300-305

[23] Addington D, Addington J, Maticka-Tyndale S. Assessing depression in schizophrenia: The Calgary depression scale. The British Journal of Psychiatry. 1993;**163**(Suppl. 22):39-44. DOI: 10.1192/S0007125000292581

[24] Lingjaerde O, Ahlfors UG, Bech P, Dencker J, Elgen K. The UKU side effect rating scale. A new comprehensive rating scale for psychotropic drugs and a cross-sectional study of side effects in neuroleptic treated patients. Acta Psychiatrica Scandinavica. 1987;**76**:1-100. DOI: 10.1111/j.1600-0447.1987.tb10566.x

[25] Pedersen IN, Bonde LO, Hannibal NJ, Nielsen J, Aagaard J, Bertelsen LR, et al. Music therapy as treatment of negative symptoms for adult patients diagnosed with schizophrenia-study protocol for a randomized, controlled and blinded study. Medicine. 2019;**646**:46. DOI: 10.3390/medicines6020046

[26] Gold C, Solli HP, Krüger V, Lie SA. Dose-response effect for music therapy for people with serious mental disturbances. Systematic review and meta-analysis. Clinical Psychology Review. 2009;**29**:193-207

[27] Simonsen E, Lyse HG, Hansen AO, Knudsen P. Om Og Med Psykoser. (About Psychosis). Copenhagen: The Psychiatry Foundation's publishing house, PsykiatriFondens Forlag; 2001

[28] Wärja M, Bonde LO. Music as co-therapist: Towards a taxonomy of music in therapeutic music and imagery work. Music and Medicine. 2014;**6**:16-27

[29] Lund HN, Pedersen IN, Johnsen SP, Heymann-Szlachcinska A, Tuszewska M, Bizik H, et al. Music to improve sleep quality in adults with depression-related insomnia (MUSTAFI): Study protocol for a randomized controlled trial. Trials. 2020;**21**(1):1-10

Section 4

Pharmacotherapy

Chapter 5

Sex Differences in and Pharmacotherapy of Schizophrenia

Norio Yasui-Furukori, Ryota Yoshida and Kazutaka Shimoda

Abstract

Schizophrenia is a common disorder with a prevalence rate of approximately 1%; its symptoms primarily of consist of positive and negative symptoms as well as cognitive decline. Moreover, sex differences are present in schizophrenia. The age of onset differs between men and women, but other sex differences occur in the symptoms, severity, number of treatments, and suicide rates. Important sex differences in the treatment of schizophrenia include the use of antipsychotic pharmacokinetics, side effects such as metabolic abnormalities, cardiovascular disease, QT prolongation, and gonadal dysfunction, and safety during pregnancy and lactation. Sex differences in antipsychotic side effects have not been fully investigated, but some have been reported to be worse in women. This article outlines sex differences in pharmacokinetics, side effects such as metabolic abnormalities, cardiovascular disease, QT prolongation, gonadal dysfunction, and pregnancy and lactation, as well as the precautions for each antipsychotic.

Keywords: schizophrenia, sex differences, antipsychotics, pharmacokinetics, side effects

1. Introduction

Schizophrenia is a common disorder with a prevalence of approximately 1% and mainly consists of positive symptoms (such as delusions and hallucinations), negative symptoms (such as decreased motivation and flat affect), and cognitive decline. Clinical observations have shown sex differences in some psychiatric disorders, including schizophrenia, but the etiology of sex differences in schizophrenia is only partially understood.

Men and women with schizophrenia have been suggested to experience differential disease progression, including age of onset, symptoms, severity, and number of treatments [1]. Men have an earlier age of onset than women, with the average age of onset ranging from 18 to 25 years for men and 25 to 35 years for women [2]; a second peak occurs in women after the age of 40 [3]. In terms of symptoms, men tend to have more negative symptoms and more severe clinical features, especially social withdrawal and substance abuse (of alcohol, nicotine, marijuana, stimulants, etc.). On the other hand, women are more likely to exhibit mood disorders and depressive symptoms as well as affective symptoms. In general, women have a better prognosis than men, with less frequent hospitalization, lower suicide rates, and better relationships with family and friends. Whether these differences are due to sex differences in response to antipsychotic treatment is not well understood, and there are currently no consistent treatment guidelines according to sex. Additionally, sex differences in antipsychotic side effects have not been fully investigated, although some side effects have been reported to be particularly problematic for women.

This article outlines the sex differences in pharmacokinetics, side effects (metabolic abnormalities, cardiovascular disease, QT prolongation, and gonadal dysfunction), and pregnancy and lactation, as well as the precautions for each antipsychotic.

2. Pharmacokinetics in women

Women reportedly experience side effects from more drugs than men, but it is not clear whether this is due to sex differences in drug pharmacokinetics and pharmacodynamics. Changes in pharmacokinetics are thought to play a major role in the efficacy and safety of drug therapy in women. Hormonal influences on physiological function may result in differences in drug absorption, protein binding, distribution volume, and metabolism in women. Sex differences have also been observed in phase I (cytochrome P450) and phase II (especially glucuronide conjugation) responses. In addition, women have a higher percentage of body fat than men, which results in a longer half-life and accumulation of lipophilic antipsychotics. This suggests that longer dosing periods are needed, especially during pregnancy [4]. Furthermore, differences in drug distribution between males and females have been attributed to differences in body size. Differences in hepatic enzyme activity are also believed to play a major role in determining sex differences in pharmacokinetics; CYP3A4, CYP2D6, and CYP1A2 are the most important enzymes in the hepatic metabolism of antipsychotic drugs [5]. Data on potential sex differences in cytochrome (CYP) activity indicate that in women, CYP3A4 and CYP2D6 activity is higher in women, especially during pregnancy and premenopause. On the other hand, CYP1A2, CYP2C19, CYP2E1, and phase II glucuronyltransferases are less active in women. These differences in enzyme activity may result in greater sex differences in plasma concentrations, leading to different clinical outcomes in men and women [6]. In some studies, plasma concentrations of clozapine and olanzapine are higher in women, possibly due to lower CYP1A2 activity [7]. The individual-level factors with the greatest influence on olanzapine pharmacokinetics are sex and smoking status [8]. For example, a young male patient with a history of smoking requires an olanzapine dose three to four times higher to reach the same plasma concentration as an elderly female patient with no smoking history [7]. However, no sex differences in plasma concentrations of risperidone, ziprasidone, quetiapine, or aripiprazole have been found. Furthermore, the renal clearance of drugs that are not actively secreted and reabsorbed is dependent on the glomerular filtration rate, which is directly proportional to body weight and is therefore higher, on average, in men than in women. Most sex differences in renal excretion rates are thought to be due to simple weight differences [9]. In summary, an awareness of the pharmacokinetics of sex differences may provide clues for appropriate drug selection and drug dosage decisions.

3. Sex differences in the risk of antipsychotic-induced metabolic abnormalities and cardiovascular disease

Women have often been excluded from large cardiovascular clinical trials in the past, but in recent years, a vast amount of accumulated data has led to the optimization of cardiovascular health in female patients by addressing sex-specific health issues [10]. Cardiovascular disease (CVD) is the leading cause of death in patients with schizophrenia, resulting in lifespans up to 30 years shorter in patients with schizophrenia compared to the general population [11]. Antipsychotic use increases the risk of certain metabolic abnormalities and may increase the risk of CVD [12]. In particular, second-generation antipsychotics cause obesity (especially abdominal obesity) due to weight gain, dyslipidemia (hypercholesterolemia, hypertriglyceridemia, hypo-high-density lipoproteinemia [hypo-HDLemia], and hyper-low-density lipoproteinemia [hyperLDLemia]), and glucose homeostasis disorders (hyperglycemia, insulin resistance, and type 2 diabetes). Up to 50% of patients receiving second-generation antipsychotics meet the criteria for metabolic syndrome, significantly increasing CVD morbidity and mortality [13]. The results of Clinical Antipsychotic Trials of Intervention Effectiveness (CATIE), a large clinical trial of antipsychotics, showed a higher prevalence and risk of metabolic syndrome in women than in men [14]. In particular, a higher incidence of metabolic syndrome was reported in patients receiving clozapine and olanzapine [15], suggesting that the risk of metabolic syndrome and CVD is very high in women receiving these drugs. On the other hand, there are also reports of elevated total cholesterol and LDL in women taking clozapine and olanzapine, whereas men have the highest risk of low HDL [16]. The above findings should be kept in mind when prescribing antipsychotic medications, and the risks and benefits should be considered. It is also important to conduct preventive screening, such as blood tests, at least once a year for men and every 6 months for women, with the goal of reducing the risk of metabolic abnormalities.

4. Sex differences in the effect of antipsychotics on the corrected QT (QTc) interval

The QT interval is defined as the interval between the beginning of the Q wave and the end of the T wave on the electrocardiogram (ECG) and is a measure of the duration of the action potential of ventricular muscle or the time from the start of depolarization to the end of repolarization. Studies in humans have shown that a prolonged QT interval increases the risk of developing torsades de pointes, a hyperplastic ventricular disease leading to ventricular fibrillation and sudden death [17]. According to a meta-analysis, women accounted for 70% of the 332 cases of torsade de pointes, but the proportion of cardiovascular drugs used in these cases was only 44%. A higher than expected incidence of torsades de pointes in women was consistently observed for all cardiovascular drugs analyzed [18]. In clinical and experimental studies, being female is associated with a longer baseline QTc interval and greater responsiveness to drugs that block cardiac voltage-dependent potassium channels, both of which increase arrhythmia induction [19]. Antipsychotics are associated with prolongation of the QT interval, which can lead to ventricular arrhythmias and sudden death [20]. First-generation antipsychotics are associated with a higher risk of QTc interval prolongation than second-generation antipsychotics [21]; however, one retrospective cohort study reported a twofold increased risk of sudden cardiac death from taking quetiapine, olanzapine, and risperidone, which was attributed to prolongation of the QT interval [22]. Aripiprazole is better tolerated than other antipsychotics with respect to its side effects, including QT prolongation, but its exact effects on the QT interval remain unknown [23]. A study conducted in Japan reported that olanzapine and quetiapine treatment had a greater impact on the

QTc interval than risperidone and aripiprazole and that these effects were particularly pronounced in female subjects [24]. As noted above, healthy women have longer QT intervals than healthy men [25], and female sex is known to be a risk factor for QTc interval prolongation [25]. Sex hormones are a major factor affecting the length of the QT interval, and estrogen has been suggested to prolong the QT interval due to bradycardia. Moreover, studies have reported a negative correlation between body mass index (BMI) and the QTc interval in women taking antipsychotics [24], which is thought to be due to decreased plasma concentrations of antipsychotics associated with increased drug distribution. In light of the above, if an individual exhibits risk factors for QT interval prolongation, such as being female or having a low BMI, it is necessary to take sex differences into account when considering the effect of each antipsychotic on the QTc interval to select an appropriate drug.

5. Antipsychotic-induced gonadal dysfunction

Gonadal dysfunction is common in patients with schizophrenia and leads to decreased quality of life and drug adherence [26]. Many studies have reported that psychiatric disorders are not the cause of gonadal dysfunction; instead, the cause is suspected to be the administration of antipsychotic medications [27]. In contrast, reports have indicated that mental illness itself is a risk factor [28]. Of the individuals treated with antipsychotic drugs, it is estimated that more than 50% of men and 30% of women experience gonadal dysfunction [29]. The most common side effects include erectile dysfunction, ejaculation problems, orgasm disorders, and decreased sexual interest in men; in women, the most common side effects are amenorrhea, dysmenorrhea, orgasm disorders, and decreased sexual interest. The most common side effects reported by men and women are erectile dysfunction in men and decreased sexual interest in women [30]. Patient distress due to these side effects is also reported to be greater in men [31]. There is no apparent relationship between the duration of treatment and gonadal dysfunction [32]. However, a higher incidence of sexual dysfunction is associated with the use of typical antipsychotics compared to atypical antipsychotics [33]. These side effects may be caused by anticholinergic effects, alpha1 adrenergic receptor inhibition, or hyperprolactinemia [34]. A study that evaluated sexual dysfunction in 101 patients receiving typical antipsychotics reported a relationship between prolactin levels and sexual dysfunction in both men and women [33]. In contrast to other atypical antipsychotics, risperidone causes a sustained increase in prolactin levels [35]. While there are reports of no significant differences in gonadal dysfunction among antipsychotics [36] significant differences have been shown between olanzapine and risperidone [30]. One study reported that olanzapine modification improved hyperprolactinemia and reduced sexual dysfunction in female schizophrenic patients treated with risperidone [37]. Additionally, relatively low rates of gonadal dysfunction are reported with quetiapine [30]. Thus, the prevalence of gonadal dysfunction in schizophrenic patients is high, the resulting decrease in drug adherence is a concern, and drug modification should be considered if necessary.

6. Antipsychotics during pregnancy and lactation

The risks of treatment with antipsychotics during pregnancy or lactation must be evaluated separately for the mother and child, comparing the risk of untreated maternal disease with the risk of toxic effects on the mother and child. One study reported that alterations in drug metabolism occur during pregnancy, with decreased CYP1A2 activity and increased CYP2D6 and CYP3A activity. Drug adjustment during pregnancy depends on the drug and the enzyme responsible for metabolism. Atypical antipsychotics have not demonstrated a clear advantage in safety during pregnancy or lactation compared to typical antipsychotics [38]. Olanzapine, risperidone, quetiapine, and clozapine do not increase the risk of fetal teratogenicity, but the use of aripiprazole, amisulpride, and ziprasidone is undesirable. However, several case reports have documented the development of gestational diabetes in women treated with clozapine or olanzapine during pregnancy. Clozapine is not recommended for use during pregnancy because it can cause floppy infant syndrome, neonatal seizures [39], gestational diabetes associated with shoulder dystocia in newborns [40], and agranulocytosis in newborns. During breastfeeding, infant drug exposure is generally less than 10% of the mother's dose. Plasma concentrations of olanzapine and risperidone in infants are also very low and may be below the detection limit [41], and quetiapine has been reported to be ingested at very low doses of 0.09% of the weight-adjusted maternal dose [42]. In contrast, clozapine tends to accumulate in infant serum, and concentrations in breast milk are relatively high and should be avoided [43].

7. Conclusion

This review has outlined sex differences in pharmacotherapy for schizophrenia. In addition to the sex differences described here, many studies are currently investigating others. In clinical practice, however, treatment based on sex differences has not yet become widespread, and both men and women are treated almost identically. Psychiatric disorders, in particular, are likely to be chronic and require long-term intervention. Therefore, it can be inferred that the importance of sex-specific medical care tailored to the characteristics of each patient will increase in the future.

Conflict of interest

The all authors have no relationships with companies or organizations that would result in conflicts of interest that should be disclosed.

Author details

Norio Yasui-Furukori*, Ryota Yoshida and Kazutaka Shimoda
Department of Neuropsychiatry, Dokkyo Medical University School of Medicine, Mibu, Tochigi, Japan

*Address all correspondence to: furukori@dokkyomed.ac.jp

References

[1] Nawka A, Kalisova L, Raboch J, Giacco D, Cihal L, Onchev G, et al. Gender differences in coerced patients with schizophrenia. BMC Psychiatry. 2013;**13**:257. DOI: 10.1186/1471-244X-13-257

[2] Häfner H, Maurer K, Löffler W, Fätkenheuer B, van der Heiden W, Riecher-Rössler A, et al. The epidemiology of early schizophrenia. Influence of age and gender on onset and early course. The British Journal of Psychiatry. Supplement. 1994;**23**:29-38

[3] Castle DJ, Wessely S, Murray RM. Sex and schizophrenia: Effects of diagnostic stringency, and associations with and premorbid variables. The British Journal of Psychiatry. 1993;**162**:658-664. DOI: 10.1192/bjp.162.5.658

[4] Pollck BG. Gender differences in psychotropic drug metabolism. Psychopharmacology Bulletin. 1997;**33**(2):235-241

[5] Prior TI, Baker GB. Interactions between the cytochrome P450 system and second-generation antipsychotics. Journal of Psychiatry & Neuroscience. 2003;**28**(2):99-112

[6] Anthony M, Berg MJ. Biologic and molecular mechanisms for sex. Differences in pharmacokinetics, pharmacodynamics, and pharmacogenetics: Part II. Journal of Women's Health & Gender-Based Medicine. 2002;**11**(7):617-629. DOI: 10.1089/152460902760360568

[7] Gex-Fabry M, Balant-Gorgia AE, Balant LP. Therapeutic drug monitoring of olanzapine: The combined effect of age, gender, smoking, and comedication. Therapeutic Drug Monitoring. 2003;**25**(1):46-53. DOI: 10.1097/00007691-200302000-00007

[8] Callaghan JT, Bergstrom RF, Ptak LR, Beasley CM. Olanzapine: Pharmacokinetic and pharmacodynamics profile. Clinical Pharmacokinetics. 1999;**37**(3):177-193. DOI: 10.2165/00003088-199937030-00001

[9] Meibohm B, Beierle I, Derendorf H. How important are dender differences in pharmacokinetics? Clinical Pharmacokinetics. 2002;**41**(5):329-342. DOI: 10.2165/00003088-200241050-00002

[10] Collins P, Steavenson JC, Mosca L. Spotlight on gender. Cardiovascular Research. 2002;**53**(3):535-537. DOI: 10.1016/s0008-6363(02)00224-9

[11] Colton CW, Manderscheid RW. Congruencies in increased mortality rates, years of potential life lost, and causes of death among public mental health. Preventing Chronic Disease. 2006;**3**(2):A42

[12] Newcomer JW. Second-generation (atypical) antipsychotics and metabolic effects: A comprehensive literature review. CNS Drugs. 2005;**19**(Suppl. 1):1-93. DOI: 10.2165/00023210-200519001-00001

[13] Meyer JM, Koro CE. The effects of antipsychotic therapy on serum lipids: A comprehensive review. Schizophrenia Research. 2004;**70**(1):1-17. DOI: 10.1016/j.schres.2004.01.014

[14] McEvoy JP, Meyer JM, Goff DC, Nasrallah HA, Davis SM, Sullivan L, et al. Prevalence of the metabolic syndrome in patients with schizophrenia: Baseline results from the clinical

antipsychotic trials of intervention effectiveness (CATIE) schizophrenia trial and comparison with national estimates from NHANES III. Schizophrenia Research. 2005;**80**(1):19-32. DOI: 10.1016/j.schres.2005.07.014

[15] Hägg S, Lindblom Y, Mjörndal T, Adolfsson R. High prevalence of the metabolic syndrome among a Swedish cohort of patients with schizophrenia. International Clinical Psychopharmacology. 2006;**21**(2):93-98. DOI: 10.1097/01.yic.0000188215.84784.17

[16] Kraal AZ, Ward KM, Ellingrod VL. Sex differences in antipsychotic related metabolic functioning in schizophrenia Spectrum disorders. Psychopharmacology Bulletin. 2017;**47**(2):8-21

[17] Haddad PM, Anderson IM. Antipsychotic-related QTc prolongation, torsade de pointes and sudden death. Drugs. 2002;**62**(11):1649-1671. DOI: 10.2165/00003495-200262110-00006

[18] Larsen JA, Kadish AH. Effects of gender on cardiac arrhythmias. Journal of Cardiovascular Electrophysiology. 1998;**9**(6):655-664. DOI: 10.1111/j.1540-8167.1998.tb00950.x

[19] Drici MD, Clement N. Is gender a risk factor for adverse drug reactions? The example of drug-induced long QT syndrome. Drug Safety. 2001;**24**(8):575-585. DOI: 10.2165/00002018-200124080-00002

[20] Glassman AH, Bigger JT. Antipsychotic drugs: Prolonged QTc interval, torsade de pointes, and sudden death. The American Journal of Psychiatry. 2001;**158**(11):1774-1782. DOI: 10.1176/appi.ajp.158.11.1774

[21] Vieweg WV. New generation antipsychotic drugs and QTc interval prolongation. Prim Care Companion to the Journal of Clinical Psychiatry. 2003;**5**(5):205-215. DOI: 10.4088/pcc.v05n0504

[22] Ray WA, Chung CP, Murray KT, Hall K, Stein CM. Atypical antipsychotic drugs and the risk of sudden cardiac death. The New England Journal of Medicine. 2009;**360**(3):225-235. DOI: 10.1056/NEJMoa0806994

[23] Pigott TA, Carson WH, Saha AR, Torbeyns AF, Stock EG, Ingenito GG. Aripiprazole study group: Aripiprazole for the prevention of relapse in stabilized patients with chronic schizophrenia: A placebo-controlled 26-week study. The Journal of Clinical Psychiatry. 2003;**64**(9):1048-1056. DOI: 10.4088/jcp.v64n0910

[24] Suzuki Y, Sugai T, Fukui N, Watanabe J, Ono S, Tsuneyama N, et al. Sex differences in the effect of four second-generation antipsychotics on QTc interval in patients. Human Psychopharmacology. 2013;**28**(3):215-219. DOI: 10.1002/hup.2309

[25] Kotin J, Wilbert DE, Verburg D, Soldinger SM. Thioridazine and sexual dysfunction. The American Journal of Psychiatry. 1976;**133**(1):82-85. DOI: 10.1176/ajp.133.1.82

[26] Olfson M, Uttaro T, Carson WH, Tafesse E. Male sexual dysfunction and quality of life in schizophrenia. The Journal of Clinical Psychiatry. 2005;**66**(3):331-338. DOI: 10.4088/jcp.v66n0309

[27] Gopalakrishnan R, Jacob KS, Kuruvilla A, Vasantharaj B, John JK. Sildenafil in the treatment of antipsychotic-induced erectile dysfunction: A randomized. The American Journal of Psychiatry. 2006;**163**(3):494-499. DOI: 10.1176/appi.ajp.163.3.494

[28] Aizenberg D, Zemishlany Z, Dorfman-Etrog P, Weizman A. Sexual dysfunction in male schizophrenic patients. The Journal of Clinical Psychiatry. 1995;**56**(4):137-141

[29] Ghadirian AM, Chouinard G, Annable L. Sexual dysfunction and plasma prolactin levels in neuroleptic-treated schizophrenic outpatients. The Journal of Nervous and Mental Disease. 1982;**170**(8):463-467. DOI: 10.1097/00005053-198208000-00004

[30] Bobes J, Garc A-Portilla MP, Rejas J, Hern Ndez G, Garcia-Garcia M, Rico-Villademoros F, et al. Frequency of sexual dysfunction and other reproductive side-effects in patients with schizophrenia. Journal of Sex & Marital Therapy. 2003;**29**(2):125-147. DOI: 10.1080/713847170

[31] Fakhoury WK, Wright D, Wallace M. Prevalence and extent of distress of adverse effects of antipsychotics among callers to a United Kingdom National Mental Health Helpline. International Clinical Psychopharmacology. 2001;**16**(3):153-162. DOI: 10.1097/00004850-200105000-00004

[32] Lingjaerde O, Ahlfors UG, Bech P, Dencker SJ, Elgen K. The UKU side effect rating scale. A new comprehensive rating scale for psychotropic drugs and a cross-sectional study of side effects in neuroleptic-treated patients. Acta Psychiatrica Scandinavica. Supplementum. 1987;**334**:1-100. DOI: 10.1111/j.1600-0447.1987.tb10566.x

[33] Smith SM, O'Keane V, Murray R. Sexual dysfunction in patients taking conventional antipsychotic medication. The British Journal of Psychiatry. 2002;**181**:49-55. DOI: 10.1192/bjp.181.1.49

[34] DeBusk R, Drory Y, Goldstein I, Jackson G, Kaul S, Kimmel SE, et al. Management of sexual dysfunction in patients with cardiovascular disease: Recommendations of the Princeton consensus panel. The American Journal of Cardiology. 2000;**86**(2):175-181. DOI: 10.1016/s0002-9149(00)00896-1

[35] Huang ML, Van Peer A, Woestenborghs R, De Coster R, Heykants J, Jansen AA, et al. Pharmacokinetics of the novel antipsychotic agent risperidone and the prolactin response in healthy. Clinical Pharmacology and Therapeutics. 1993;**54**(3):257-268. DOI: 10.1038/clpt.1993.146

[36] Fujii A, Yasui-Furukori N, Sugawara N, Sato Y, Nakagami T, Saito M, et al. Sexual dysfunction in Japanese patients with schizophrenia treated with antipsychotics. Progress in Neuro-Psychopharmacology & Biological Psychiatry. 2010;**34**(2):288-293. DOI: 10.1016/j.pnpbp.2009.11.022

[37] Kim KS, Pae CU, Chae JH, Bahk WM, Jun TY, Kim DJ, et al. Effects of olanzapine on prolactin levels of female patients with schizophrenia treated with risperidone. The Journal of Clinical Psychiatry. 2002;**63**(5):408-413. DOI: 10.4088/jcp.v63n0506

[38] Gentile S. Clinical utilization of atypical antipsychotics in pregnancy and lactation. The Annals of Pharmacotherapy. 2004;**38**(7-8):1265-1271. DOI: 10.1345/aph.1D485

[39] Stoner SC, Sommi RW Jr, Marken PA, Anya I, Vaughn J. Clozapine use in two full-term pregnancies. The Journal of Clinical Psychiatry. 1997;**58**(8):364-365. DOI: 10.4088/jcp.v58n0806f

[40] Dickson RA, Hogg L. Pregnancy of a patient treated with clozapine. Psychiatric Services.

1998;**49**(8):1081-1083. DOI: 10.1176/ps.49.8.1081

[41] Aichhorn W, Stuppaeck C, Whitworth AB. Risperidone and breast-feeding. Journal of Psychopharmacology. 2005;**19**(2):211-213. DOI: 10.1177/0269881105049044

[42] Lee A, Giesbrecht E, Dunn E, Ito S. Excretion of quetiapine in breast milk. The American Journal of Psychiatry. 2004;**161**(9):1715-1716. DOI: 10.1176/appi.ajp.161.9.1715-a

[43] Bennett JA, Keck PE. A target-dose finding study of clozapine in patients with schizophrenia. Annals of Clinical Psychiatry. 1996;**8**(1):19-21. DOI: 10.3109/10401239609149086

Section 5

Clinical and Biology

Chapter 6

Clinical and Biological Overlap between Schizophrenia, Autism Spectrum Disorder, and Trauma and Stress-Related Disorders: The Three-Tree Model of SCZ-ASD-TSRD

Hitomi Shimizu, Yoshiro Morimoto, Naoki Yamamoto, Hirokazu Kumazaki, Hiroki Ozawa and Akira Imamura

Abstract

There is significant overlap in the clinical and neurobiological profiles of schizophrenia (SCZ), autism spectrum disorder (ASD), and trauma- and stress-related disorders (TSRDs); moreover, they often co-occur as comorbid disorders. Although current international classification criteria and those in the psychiatry/psychology field recognize such comorbidities, the assessment and treatment of these patients are provided as independent disorders. In this chapter, we summarize the current understanding of the attributes shared by the three disorders and discuss the possible contributors to the development of SCZ, ASD, and TSRD, which include environmental, genetic, and biological factors. We also propose a three-tree model that represents the clinical and biological relationships among the three diseases as a new perspective for assessing and treating these disorders. A comprehensive understanding of these disorders will enable improvements in medical care for patients with these illnesses.

Keywords: schizophrenia, autism spectrum disorder, trauma- and stress-related disorders, adverse childhood experiences, psychiatric disorder

1. Introduction

Schizophrenia (SCZ) is a severe chronic neuropsychiatric disorder characterized by a mixture of positive and negative symptoms. Positive symptoms reflect cognitive excesses or errors (e.g. delusions, hallucinations, and disorganized behaviors), whereas negative symptoms reflect a decrease or absence of normal behaviors (e.g. avoidance, loss of pleasure, and asociality) and expressions (e.g. insensitive emotions and alogia) that depend on motivation and interest [1]. Patients with SCZ are usually

IntechOpen

treated with antipsychotic medications; however, approximately 30% of cases are unresponsive to drug treatment and are referred to as having treatment-resistant SCZ (TRS) [2]. Owing to these distinctive clinical aspects of the chronic and severe disease course, SCZ is considered a global burden [3].

Several psychiatric disorders present with similar clinical symptoms to those of SCZ, and the differentiation and comorbidity of these disorders with SCZ is a common clinical problem. Autism spectrum disorder (ASD) is a neurodevelopmental disorder, and core symptoms include impairments in social interactions and communication and the presence of restricted and repetitive behaviors [4]. Notably, it has recently become widely recognized in clinical practice that some of the symptoms of SCZ (especially negative symptoms) and ASD share similarities [4]. Trauma- and stress-related disorders (TSRDs) are a group of emotional and behavioral problems that result from childhood trauma and stress experiences, which have also received attention as disorders that exhibit symptoms similar to those of SCZ, especially the positive symptoms of SCZ [5]. Traumatic and stressful experiences that cause TSRD include exposure to physical and emotional violence and distress, such as abuse and neglect.

It is well established that SCZ, ASD, and TSRD often co-occur as comorbid disorders. Such comorbidities are recognized in international classification criteria for psychiatric disorders, such as the Diagnostic and Statistical Manual of Mental Disorders Fifth Edition (DSM-5) and the International Classification of Diseases, 11th Revision (ICD-11) [6, 7]; moreover, the comorbidity of these disorders is widely recognized by professionals in the clinical psychiatry field (e.g. psychiatrists and clinical psychologists). However, the assessment and treatment of patients with these disorders are independent of each other, and the importance of comprehensively understanding and assessing these disorders is not widely recognized. The purpose of this chapter is to summarize recent research findings on the clinical, epidemiological, and biological correlates of SCZ, ASD, and TSRD and provide new perspectives on providing better medical care for patients with SCZ.

2. History of the debate on the relationship between SCZ, ASD, and childhood living environment

The term SCZ was first coined by Eugen Bleuler in 1908 and stems from the Greek words "schizo" (split) and "phren" (mind) [8]. Bleuler categorized the clinical symptoms of SCZ into basic, primary, and secondary symptoms. The basic symptoms are known as the famous Bleuler's four As: alogia, autism, ambivalence, and affect blunting [9]. Schneider's 1939 proposal of "first-rank symptoms" (FRSs) was incorporated into the SCZ section of the DSM-III and has greatly influenced the diagnostic approaches for SCZ for several decades [10].

In 1943, Leo Kanner reported detailed observations on 11 cases of children with "autistic disturbances of emotional contact" [11], who were described as having "infantile autism," based on the symptoms of "autism" that Bleuler had previously described as typical symptoms of adult patients with SCZ. Kanner also described "autism" as independent of SCZ and explained that autism is not a precursor to SCZ and that autism symptoms are evident immediately after birth or in early childhood [10]. However, during this time, "infancy autism" was generally considered the earliest form of childhood SCZ; that is, a subtype of SCZ. In the late 1960s, Rutter introduced the notion that infancy autism is a developmental disorder rather than

SCZ by questioning the view that infancy autism and SCZ are the same disorder given their differences, such as the age of onset [12, 13]. Wing defined impairments in interpersonal interactions as impairments in interpersonal cognition, interpersonal communication, and interpersonal imagination and understanding, and referred to these symptoms as a continuum of autistic traits [14]. Wing broadened Kanner and Rutter's concepts of autism to include a wider range of symptoms [15], which subsequently became the basis for the current definition of ASD and, in turn, contributed to the development of a more comprehensive disease concept of neurodevelopmental disorders. Therefore, since the disease concept was established, it was assumed that ASD symptoms would overlap with those of SCZ.

The association between SCZ and ASD and an inappropriate nurturing environment was discussed during the early stage of establishing the disease concepts of ASD and SCZ. As early as 1943, Leo Kanner reported that mothers of autistic children lacked warmth and affection [11]. This theory that parenting attitudes lead to the development of ASD and SCZ in children is known as the "refrigerator mother" theory and was aggressively adopted by the medical community around 1950 as a label for parents of children diagnosed with autism and SCZ. However, this theory was largely refuted in the mid-1960s, and most medical professionals no longer accept this theory today. Nevertheless, extensive research on the relationship between child maltreatment (including all types of abuse and neglect of children by parents, caregivers, or other persons in custodial roles) and ASD/SCZ is ongoing, and various new findings have renewed the outdated and prejudiced "refrigerator mother" theory.

3. Clinical overlap between ASD and SCZ

Recent reports have indicated that a family history of psychiatric disorders, including SCZ, is not uncommon in families with ASD patients. In fact, 63% of ASD patients have a family history of some form of psychiatric disorder; moreover, a family history of SCZ is associated with a 2.1-fold increase in the odds ratio (ORs) for a child developing ASD [16]. Parental SCZ has been shown to be associated with an increased risk of ASD in Swedish nationals (OR = 2.9, 95% confidence interval [CI] = 2.5–3.4) and Stockholm County cohorts (OR = 2.9, 95% CI = 2.0–4.1). Similarly, an increased risk of ASD has been reported in Swedish nationals (OR = 2.6, 95% CI = 2.0–3.2) and Israeli conscript cohorts (OR = 12.1, 95% CI = 4.5–32) who have a peer with ASD [17]. It is estimated that up to 34.8% of ASD patients will be diagnosed with a psychiatric disorder in their lifetime and between 3.6% and 60% will develop SCZ [18]. Patients with ASD show deficits in social-emotional reciprocity and engagement, which include lack of emotional empathy, lack of social activity, lack of nonverbal communication, and reduced spontaneous communication and conversation [19], and clinically distinguishing between these behavioral characteristics of ASD and the negative symptoms of SCZ (which may include impairments in social communication and social and emotional interactions) is often difficult; indeed, in some cases, there is a comorbidity of the two disorders [20]. Furthermore, some patients with ASD have additional symptoms that are suggestive of comorbid psychotic disorders [21]. For example, ASD patients often present with symptoms related to language abnormalities, such as echolalia and abnormal intonation, atypical social behaviors (e.g. exaggerated gestures and facial expressions), inappropriate sociability, sensory sensitivity, repetitive hand and body movements, adherence to routinized behaviors, and stereotyped and repetitive behaviors (e.g. restricted interests), and adherence to identity [19], and differentiating between these characteristic behaviors of ASD patients and positive symptoms in SCZ is often challenging [21].

4. Clinical overlap between SCZ and TSRD

Adverse traumatic experiences, such as discrimination, social-environmental adversity, bullying, migration, and childhood trauma, can all be risk factors for mental illness, and the development of SCZ is no exception [22]. In a meta-analysis of studies published between 1806 and March 1, 2013, childhood trauma experiences were found to contribute to the development of SCZ with ORs ranging from 2.01 to 4.15 [23]. Another meta-analysis of studies published between July 2016 and July 2021 similarly found that childhood adversity experiences played a role in the development of SCZ [8]. In contrast, a systematic review published in 2012 on SCZ and adverse traumatic experiences showed that patients with psychosis were 2.72 times more likely than controls to be exposed to childhood adversity [24]. Whether childhood adversity experiences lead to the development of psychiatric disorders has been shown to be influenced by the timing and type of trauma. The probability of developing SCZ was high for those who had been exposed to several types of childhood adversity: sexual abuse (OR = 2.38, 95% CI = 1.98–2.87), physical abuse (OR = 2.95, 95% CI = 2.25–3.88), and psychological abuse (OR = 3.40, 95% CI = 2.06–5.62) [24]. There were also significant differences between all types of childhood adversity and psychiatric disorders, except parental death [24]. A review that assessed self-reported childhood experiences of SCZ patients indicated that 26% had been sexually abused, 39% had been physically abused, and 34% had been psychologically abused [25]. Additionally, it has been reported that even a single experience of sexual abuse specifically increases the probability of developing and severity of SCZ [26, 27].

Childhood trauma experiences are also associated with the degree of symptoms, with higher levels of trauma being associated with more positive symptoms, depressive symptoms, and lower levels of cognitive functioning. Childhood trauma experiences are associated more with positive symptoms, such as hallucinations and delusions, than with negative symptoms [5]. Childhood trauma induces dissociation, where stronger childhood trauma experiences are reflected by higher scores on the Dissociative Experiences Scale (DES), which measures dissociation. Positive symptoms have also been shown to correlate positively with DES scores in SCZ patients [28]. Indeed, some researchers have proposed the idea that symptoms such as hallucinations and delusions reflect a personal perception of intrusion that leads to a sense of hopelessness [5]. Furthermore, it is worth noting that the direction of Schneider's first-class symptoms, which were historically considered important symptoms of SCZ, are more common in patients with dissociative identity disorder than in those with SCZ [29]. These reports provide a valuable perspective on the importance of differentiating dissociative symptoms from the positive symptoms of SCZ. It is also of clinical importance to note that patients with both psychotic disorders and a history of childhood maltreatment have higher rates of hospitalization because of symptoms, more persistent and earlier onset of psychosis, more severe episodes, higher rates of treatment failure, and a higher risk of suicide and substance abuse [30].

As described earlier, there is accumulating evidence of a close relationship between TRS and SCZ at both diagnostic and symptomatic levels. Therefore, the importance of assessment and treatment approaches for psychotic patients who consider the presence of adverse traumatic experiences should be emphasized.

5. Clinical overlap between ASD and TSRD

Empirical research on the effects of adverse trauma in ASD patients is surprisingly limited. Mandell et al. found that out of 156 children with ASD, 18.5% had been physically abused, 16.6% had been sexually abused, and physically and sexually abused children were more likely than non-abused children to engage in sexual and abusive behaviors [31]. It was also reported in a sample of children and adolescents with ASD that 26% had a history of trauma [32]. Furthermore, a significant proportion of children with a history of institutional rearing or severe neglect exhibit autism-like patterns (quasi-autism), and a quarter of these quasi-autistic children show core features of autism that improve by the age of 11 years [33].

Therefore, in light of these reports, those performing medical assessments of children with ASD-like behavioral characteristics should consider that individuals who are not biologically vulnerable because of abuse or neglect may also exhibit autism-like symptoms and characteristics.

6. Biological mechanisms common to SCZ, ASD, and TSRD: genetic and other biological factors

In recent years, the relationship and overlap between functional psychiatric disorders (e.g. SCZ and bipolar disorder) and neurodevelopmental disorders have been reported; moreover, the idea that these disorders are a series of spectrums caused by genetic and environmental factors has been discussed [34, 35]. Recent genomic analyses support the biological association between functional psychiatric disorders and neurodevelopmental disorders, and the same genetic variant is often reported to be a risk factor for various psychiatric and neurodevelopmental disorders. Recurrent microdeletions and microduplications in a 600-kb genomic region of chromosome 16p11.2 have been implicated in childhood-onset developmental disorders, and a meta-analysis of multiple psychiatric datasets identified a significant association between 16p11.2 duplication and SCZ, bipolar disorder, and ASD [36]. The Cross-Disorder Group of the Psychiatric Genomics Consortium performed a meta-analysis of genome-wide association studies (GWASs) of five psychiatric disorders (ASD, attention-deficit hyperactivity disorder [ADHD], bipolar disorder, major depression, and SCZ) to identify specific disease-related variants common to these disorders. In the primary analysis, they found that single-nucleotide polymorphisms (SNPs) at four loci surpassed the cutoff for genome-wide significance ($p < 5 \times 10^{-8}$): regions on chromosomes 3p21 and 10q24 and SNPs within two L-type voltage-gated calcium channel subunits, CACNA1C and CACNB2 [37]. Another GWAS meta-analysis of SCZ, bipolar disorder, ASD, ADHD, and depression also reported significant enrichment of overlapping genes among different disorders [38]. The polygenic risk score (PRS) for common variants can be used to determine shared genetic risk among different disorders. The PRS in GWAS for multiple psychiatric disorders reports a strong correlation between SCZ and bipolar disorder and a weak yet significant correlation between SCZ and ASD [39].

In summary, reports suggesting a genetic link between functional psychiatric disorders, including SCZ, and neurodevelopmental disorders, including ASD, have been increasing annually. In recent years, SCZ has been considered a developmental risk factor model that encompasses both biological and social risk factors, rather than a simple neurodevelopmental disorder [40]. Interestingly, it has been reported that the molecular genetic risk state for SCZ shows an additive interaction with exposure to certain environmental factors (e.g. regular cannabis use or childhood adversity) [41]. Thus, it has been suggested that not only genetic factors but also numerous environmental factors increase the risk of developing SCZ. How does a traumatic experience affect the brain and lead to the development of SCZ?

When the body is stressed, the hypothalamus-pituitary-adrenal (HPA) axis responds, and child abuse survivors have been shown to possess an overreactive HPA system [42]. Functional changes in the HPA axis may alter many neurobiological elements, such as neurotransmitter function (e.g. dopamine), physiological responses via the autonomic nervous system, and structural and functional neural changes, all of which may increase vulnerability to the development of psychosis [43]. In addition, recent research on the association between childhood trauma and psychotic symptoms suggests immune system dysregulation as a biological mediator. A meta-analysis of recent traumatic experiences and immune system biomarkers revealed that individuals exposed to childhood trauma have significantly higher baseline peripheral blood C-reactive protein, interleukin (IL)-6, and tumor necrosis factor (TNF)-α. Furthermore, a subgroup analysis of patients who had been exposed to specific types of trauma (i.e. sexual, physical, and emotional abuse) showed that each type impacted single inflammatory markers differently. Notably, these results indicated that childhood trauma contributes to inflammatory conditions in adulthood and that the inflammatory profile is dependent on the type of trauma [44]. It has also been reported that only SCZ patients who had experienced childhood trauma had elevated levels of TNF-α and IL-6, whereas those who had not experienced trauma had cytokine levels similar to those of controls [45]. Additionally, all patients with first-episode SCZ had higher cytokine levels than controls. However, patients who have experienced childhood trauma have also been shown to have higher serum TNF-α levels than those who have not [46]. There have also been reports of increased messenger RNA expression of cytokine genes in the lymphocytes of SCZ patients [47], which may be due to epigenetic mechanisms that underlie the relationship between SCZ and childhood stress [48, 49]. Although very few studies have directly analyzed this association between childhood stress and epigenetic changes and schizophrenia at this time, epigenetic abnormalities in specific genetic loci, such as abnormal methylation of the glucocorticoid receptor 1 (GR-1) gene and long interspersed nucleotide element-1 (LINE-1), have been reported [50, 51].

7. Discussion

This chapter provided an overview of the comorbidities and clinical similarities between SCZ, ASD, and TSRD, as well as recent genetic and biological studies. Currently, SCZ, ASD, and TSRD are defined independently on the basis of their core concepts and symptoms in diagnostic and classification systems for mental disorders, such as the ICD-11 and DSM-5. However, recent studies have suggested that their clinical manifestations are similar and share several aspects in the context of their pathogeneses, as if they were three adjacent trees (**Figure 1**). Given these common clinical and biological aspects shared by these three disorders, the question of how psychiatric professionals should comprehend and assess these disorders remains.

To address this question, the issues around comorbidity among the disorders must be organized. The term "comorbidity" is typically used to describe conditions that simultaneously meet the multiple definitions of mental illness. Comorbidity is conventionally used to signify "coexisting" or "cooccurring" illnesses. However, some have argued that the definition of "comorbidity" is still immature [52]. Meghani et al. organized the concept of "comorbidity" as follows: 1) concurrent

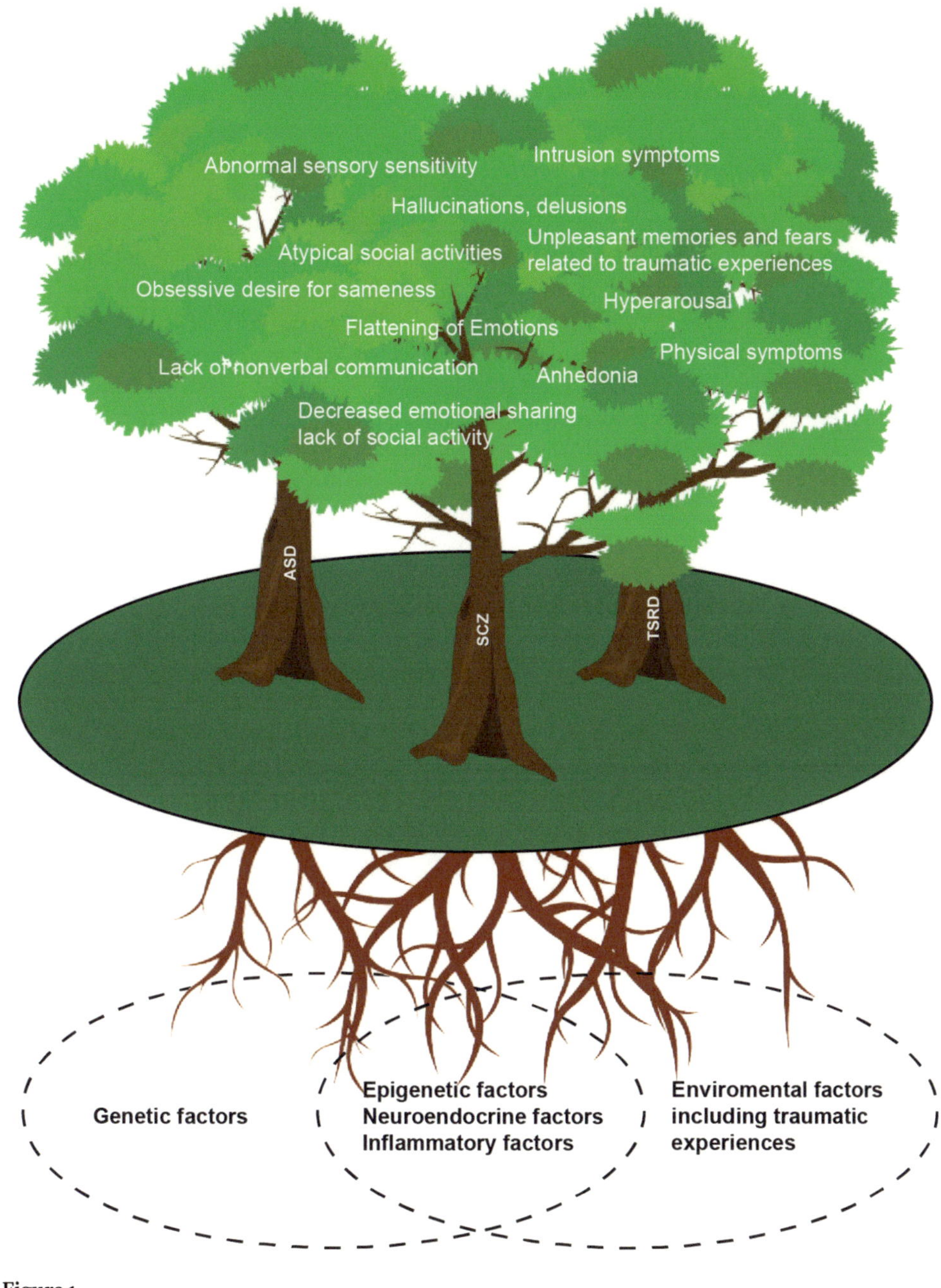

Figure 1.
The three-tree model of SCZ-ASD-TSRD. This figure represents the clinical and biological relationships among the three diseases discussed in this chapter (SCZ, ASD, and TSRD) as three trees. Although the core concepts of each disease (the tree trunk) are independent, the clinically observed symptoms (the tree crown) are shared, and the diseases share common genetic and environmental factors (including adverse traumatic experiences) that contribute to the development of the diseases. SCZ: schizophrenia, ASD: autism spectrum disorder, TSRD: trauma- and stress-related disorders.

(no "known" relationship); 2) antecedent-consequent or complicating morbidity; 3) reciprocal morbidity; 4) principal/causal morbidity (major underlying mechanism responsible for multiple diseases); and 5) latent-manifest morbidity (assumed consequent disease may have been developing slowly below the threshold level for clinical diagnosis). Of these, 1) is defined as "coexisting diseases" or "multimorbidity," and the others are defined as "cooccurring/co-dependent diseases" or "comorbidity" [52, 53]. As discussed in this chapter, there is accumulating evidence for comorbidity at both diagnostic and symptomatic levels for the three diseases; however, there remains a lack of studies that directly and empirically examine the causal relationships or mechanisms of interaction among the three diseases. Therefore, further empirical studies on the comorbidity of these diseases are essential.

In addition, recent genetic and biological analyses have provided extensive evidence for a common biological background for these diseases. This suggests that SCZ, ASD, and TSRD are not biologically independent, despite each having been given a clinically independent diagnostic category. The National Institute of Mental Health has proposed the Research Domain Criteria (RDoC) initiative to conceptualize symptoms within and across different disorders [54, 55] aimed at introducing a novel classification system that incorporates the interrelationship between the clinical phenotype of psychopathology and its underlying biological pathophysiology by dimensionally assessing and matching symptoms to several biological hierarchies, such as genetic, molecular, cellular, and neural circuitries [54, 55]. The RDoC is unique in that it explicitly focuses on the complex overlapping multidimensionality of psychiatric disorders, which allows research to be conducted without the need to consider comorbidities among disorders. In the future, research generated by the RDoC project will enable better characterization of the multidimensionality of SCZ, ASD, and TSRD and provide a basis for comprehensively understanding the three disorders.

In addition, it is worth emphasizing the utility of understanding and evaluating these three diseases comprehensively rather than as separate diseases, from the perspective of both basic and biological research, as well as clinically. For example, higher levels of dissociation have been reported in patients with TRS than in patients who are more sensitive to pharmacotherapy [56]. Furthermore, the degree of social cognitive dysfunction and autistic features in TRS patients may be similar to that in ASD patients; indeed, similarities between TRS and ASD have been reported [57]. Thus, a comprehensive assessment of ASD symptoms and traumatic experiences for patients with TRS may assist in the treatment of TRS patients. Specifically, it may be useful to assess ASD tendencies in TRS patients using standardized scales (e.g. the Autism Diagnostic Interview-Revised [ADI-R] or Autism Diagnostic Observation Schedule Second Edition [ADOS-2]) [58, 59] and traumatic experiences using structured interview (e.g. Clinician-Administered PTSD Scale for DSM-5 [CAPS-5]) [60]. In cases in whom ASD is determined to be a comorbid illness, therapeutic interventions similar to those for ASD may be effective, such as environmental adjustments that take into account communication style, lifestyle, sensory oversensitivity, under-registration, avoidance, immersion, applied behavior analysis (ABA)-based behavioral therapy, operant conditioning based on learning theory, Treatment and Education of Autistic and related Communication-handicapped Children (TEACCH), and other treatment strategies [61, 62]. Similarly, treatment strategies for TRS with comorbid TSRD may include trauma-informed care and cognitive behavioral therapy targeting the traumatic experience, which is similar to treatments for TSRD [63–65].

8. Conclusion

This chapter provided an overview of recent research findings on the clinical and biological overlap of SCZ, ASD, and TSRD. Comprehensive understanding and assessment of these disorders will not only prevent the inability to "see the forest for the trees" and provide better assessment for patients but also offer opportunities for physicians and researchers in this field to deepen their understanding of these disorders.

Acknowledgements

We thank Sarina Iwabuchi, PhD, from Edanz (www.edanz.com/ac) for editing a draft of this manuscript. This work was supported by JSPS KAKENHI (grant number 20K16650).

Conflict of interest

The authors declare no conflict of interest.

Author details

Hitomi Shimizu[1,2], Yoshiro Morimoto[1,2]*, Naoki Yamamoto[1,2], Hirokazu Kumazaki[1,2], Hiroki Ozawa[1,2] and Akira Imamura[2,3]

1 Department of Neuropsychiatry, Unit of Translational Medicine, Nagasaki University Graduate School of Biomedical Sciences, Nagasaki, Japan

2 Child and Adolescent Psychiatry Community Partnership Unit, Nagasaki University Hospital, Nagasaki, Japan

3 Department of Psychiatric Rehabilitation Science, Nagasaki University Graduate School of Biomedical Sciences, Nagasaki, Japan

*Address all correspondence to: y-morimoto@nagasaki-u.ac.jp

References

[1] Correll CU, Schooler NR. Negative symptoms in schizophrenia: A review and clinical guide for recognition, assessment, and treatment. Neuropsychiatric Disease and Treatment. 2020;**16**:519-534. DOI: 10.2147/NDT.S225643

[2] Vita A, Minelli A, Barlati S, et al. Treatment-resistant schizophrenia: Genetic and neuroimaging correlates. Frontiers in Pharmacology. 2019;**10**:402. DOI: 10.3389/fphar.2019.00402

[3] Radaic A, Martins-de-Souza D. The state of the art of nanopsychiatry for schizophrenia diagnostics and treatment. Nanomedicine. 2020;**28**:102222. DOI: 10.1016/j.nano.2020.102222

[4] Farmer C, Thurm A, Grant P. Pharmacotherapy for the core symptoms in autistic disorder: Current status of the research. Drugs. 2013;**73**(4):303-314. DOI: 10.1007/s40265-013-0021-7

[5] Inyang B, Gondal FJ, Abah GA, et al. The role of childhood trauma in psychosis and schizophrenia: A systematic review. Cureus. 2022;**14**(1):e21466. DOI: 10.7759/cureus.21466

[6] American Psychiatric Association. Diagnostic and Statistical Manual of Mental Disorders. Fifth ed. Arlington: American Psychiatric Publishing; 2013

[7] World Health Organization. ICD-11 for Mortality and Morbidity Statistics (version: 02/2022). 2022. Available from: https://icd.who.int/browse11/l-m/en

[8] Hany M, Rehman B, Azhar Y, Chapman J. Schizophrenia. Treasure Island: StatPearls Publishing; 2021

[9] Arantes-Gonçalves F, Gama Marques J, Telles-Correia D. Bleuler's psychopathological perspective on schizophrenia delusions: Towards new tools in psychotherapy treatment. Frontiers in Psychiatry. 2018;**9**:306. DOI: 10.3389/fpsyt.2018.00306

[10] Kendler KS, Mishara A. The prehistory of Schneider's first-rank symptoms: Texts from 1810 to 1932. Schizophrenia Bulletin. 2019;**45**(5):971-990. DOI: 10.1093/schbul/sbz047

[11] Kanner L. Problems of nosology and psychodynamics of early infantile autism. The American Journal of Orthopsychiatry. 1949;**19**(3):416-426. DOI: 10.1111/j.1939-0025.1949.tb05441.x

[12] Rutter M. The development of infantile autism. Psychological Medicine. 1974;**4**(2):147-163. DOI: 10.1017/s0033291700041982

[13] Rutter M. Diagnosis and definition of childhood autism. Journal of Autism and Childhood Schizophrenia. 1978;**8**(2):139-161. DOI: 10.1007/BF01537863

[14] Wing L. The continuum of autistic characteristics. In: Schopler E, Mesibov GB, editors. Diagnosis and Assessment in Autism. New York: Plenum Press; 1988. pp. 91-110. DOI: 10.1007/978-1-4899-0792-9_7

[15] Wing L. Asperger's syndrome: A clinical account. Psychological Medicine. 1981;**11**(1):115-129. DOI: 10.1017/s0033291700053332

[16] Xie S, Karlsson H, Dalman C, et al. Family history of mental and neurological disorders and risk of autism. JAMA Network Open.

2019;**2**(3):e190154. DOI: 10.1001/jamanetworkopen.2019.0154

[17] Sullivan PF, Magnusson C, Reichenberg A, et al. Family history of schizophrenia and bipolar disorder as risk factors for autism. Archives of General Psychiatry. 2012;**69**(11):1099-1103. DOI: 10.1001/archgenpsychiatry.2012.730

[18] Chisholm K, Lin A, Abu-Akel A, Wood SJ. The association between autism and schizophrenia spectrum disorders: A review of eight alternate models of co-occurrence. Neuroscience and Biobehavioral Reviews. 2015;**55**:173-183. DOI: 10.1016/j.neubiorev.2015.04.012

[19] Foss-Feig JH, McPartland JC, Anticevic A, Wolf J. Re-conceptualizing ASD within a dimensional framework: Positive, negative, and cognitive feature clusters. Journal of Autism and Developmental Disorders. 2016;**46**(1):342-351. DOI: 10.1007/s10803-015-2539-x

[20] Konstantareas MM, Hewitt T. Autistic disorder and schizophrenia: Diagnostic overlaps. Journal of Autism and Developmental Disorders. 2001;**31**(1):19-28. DOI: 10.1023/A:1005605528309

[21] Cochran DM, Dvir Y, Frazier JA. "Autism-plus" spectrum disorders: Intersection with psychosis and the schizophrenia spectrum. Child and Adolescent Psychiatric Clinics of North America. 2013;**22**(4):609-627. DOI: 10.1016/j.chc.2013.04.005

[22] Kosteletos I, Kollias K, Stefanis N. Childhood adverse traumatic experiences and schizophrenia. Psychiatriki. 2020;**31**(1):23-35

[23] Velikonja T, Fisher HL, Mason O, Johnson S. Childhood trauma and schizotypy: A systematic literature review. Psychological Medicine. 2015;**45**(5):947-963. DOI: 10.1017/S0033291714002086

[24] Varese F, Smeets F, Drukker M, et al. Childhood adversities increase the risk of psychosis: A meta-analysis of patient-control, prospective- and cross-sectional cohort studies. Schizophrenia Bulletin. 2012;**38**(4):661-671. DOI: 10.1093/schbul/sbs050

[25] Bonoldi I, Simeone E, Rocchetti M, et al. Prevalence of self-reported childhood abuse in psychosis: A meta-analysis of retrospective studies. Psychiatry Research. 2013;**210**(1):8-15. DOI: 10.1016/j.psychres.2013.05.003

[26] Mall S, Platt JM, Temmingh H, et al. The relationship between childhood trauma and schizophrenia in the Genomics of Schizophrenia in the Xhosa people (SAX) study in South Africa. Psychological Medicine. 2020;**50**(9):1570-1577. DOI: 10.1017/S0033291719001703

[27] Wickham S, Bentall R. Are specific early-life adversities associated with specific symptoms of psychosis?: A patient study considering just world beliefs as a mediator. The Journal of Nervous and Mental Disease. 2016;**204**(8):606-613. DOI: 10.1097/NMD.0000000000000511

[28] Uyan TT, Baltacioglu M, Hocaoglu C. Relationships between childhood trauma and dissociative, psychotic symptoms in patients with schizophrenia: A case-control study. Genetics Psychiatric. 2022;**35**(1):e100659. DOI: 10.1136/gpsych-2021-100659

[29] Laddis A, Dell PF. Dissociation and psychosis in dissociative identity disorder and schizophrenia. Journal of Trauma & Dissociation.

2012;**13**(4):397-413. DOI: 10.1080/15299732.2012.664967

[30] Kaufman J, Torbey S. Child maltreatment and psychosis. Neurobiology of Disease. 2019;**131**:104378. DOI: 10.1016/j.nbd.2019.01.015

[31] Mandell DS, Walrath CM, Manteuffel B, Sgro G, Pinto-Martin JA. The prevalence and correlates of abuse among children with autism served in comprehensive community-based mental health settings. Child Abuse & Neglect. 2005;**29**(12):1359-1372. DOI: 10.1016/j.chiabu.2005.06.006

[32] Mehtar M, Mukaddes NM. Posttraumatic stress disorder in individuals with diagnosis of autistic spectrum disorders. Research in Autism Spectrum Disorder. 2011;**5**(1):539-546

[33] Rutter M, Kreppner J, Croft C, et al. Early adolescent outcomes of institutionally deprived and non-deprived adoptees. III. Quasi-autism. Journal of Child Psychology and Psychiatry. 2007;**48**(12):1200-1207. DOI: 10.1111/j.1469-7610.2007.01792.x

[34] Craddock N, Owen MJ. The Kraepelinian dichotomy - going, going... but still not gone. The British Journal of Psychiatry. 2010;**196**(2):92-95

[35] Owen MJ. Intellectual disability and major psychiatric disorders: A continuum of neurodevelopmental causality. The British Journal of Psychiatry. 2012;**200**(4):268-269

[36] McCarthy SE, Makarov V, Kirov G, et al. Microduplications of 16p11.2 are associated with schizophrenia. Nature Genetics. 2009;**41**(11):1223-1227. DOI: 10.1038/ng.474

[37] Cross-Disorder Group of the Psychiatric Genomics Consortium. Identification of risk loci with shared effects on five major psychiatric disorders: A genome-wide analysis. Lancet. 2013;**381**(9875):1371-1379

[38] Wu Y, Cao H, Baranova A, Huang H, Li S, Cai L, et al. Multi-trait analysis for genome-wide association study of five psychiatric disorders. Translational Psychiatry. 2020;**10**(1):209

[39] Lee SH, Ripke S, Neale BM, Faraone SV, Purcell SM, Perlis RH, et al. Genetic relationship between five psychiatric disorders estimated from genome-wide SNPs. Nature Genetics. 2013;**45**(9):984-994

[40] Murray RM, Lewis SW. Is schizophrenia a neurodevelopmental disorder? British Medical Journal. 1987;**295**(6600):681-682. DOI: 10.1136/bmj.295.6600.681

[41] Guloksuz S, Pries LK, Delespaul P, et al. Examining the independent and joint effects of molecular genetic liability and environmental exposures in schizophrenia: Results from the EUGEI study. World Psychiatry. 2019;**18**(2):173-182. DOI: 10.1002/wps.20629

[42] Heim C, Newport DJ, Heit S, et al. Pituitary-adrenal and autonomic responses to stress in women after sexual and physical abuse in childhood. Journal of the American Medical Association. 2000;**284**(5):592-597. DOI: 10.1001/jama.284.5.592

[43] Read J, Perry BD, Moskowitz A, Connolly J. The contribution of early traumatic events to schizophrenia in some patients: A traumagenic neurodevelopmental model. Psychiatry. 2001;**64**(4):319-345. DOI: 10.1521/psyc.64.4.319.18602

[44] Baumeister D, Akhtar R, Ciufolini S, Pariante CM, Mondelli V. Childhood trauma and adulthood inflammation: A meta-analysis of peripheral C-reactive protein, interleukin-6 and tumour necrosis factor-α. Molecular Psychiatry. 2016;**21**(5):642-649. DOI: 10.1038/mp.2015.67

[45] Dennison U, McKernan D, Cryan J, Dinan T. Schizophrenia patients with a history of childhood trauma have a pro-inflammatory phenotype. Psychological Medicine. 2012;**42**(9):1865-1871. DOI: 10.1017/S0033291712000074

[46] Di Nicola M, Cattaneo A, Hepgul N, et al. Serum and gene expression profile of cytokines in first-episode psychosis. Brain, Behavior, and Immunity. 2013;**31**:90-95. DOI: 10.1016/j.bbi.2012.06.010

[47] Pandey GN, Ren X, Rizavi HS, Zhang H. Proinflammatory cytokines and their membrane-bound receptors are altered in the lymphocytes of schizophrenia patients. Schizophrenia Research. 2015;**164**(1-3):193-198. DOI: 10.1016/j.schres.2015.02.004

[48] Misiak B, Krefft M, Bielawski T, Moustafa AA, Sąsiadek MM, Frydecka D. Toward a unified theory of childhood trauma and psychosis: A comprehensive review of epidemiological, clinical, neuropsychological and biological findings. Neuroscience and Biobehavioral Reviews. 2017;**75**:393-406. DOI: 10.1016/j.neubiorev.2017.02.015

[49] Lavratti C, Dorneles G, Pochmann D, et al. Exercise-induced modulation of histone H4 acetylation status and cytokines levels in patients with schizophrenia. Physiology & Behavior. 2017;**168**:84-90. DOI: 10.1016/j.physbeh.2016.10.021

[50] Misiak B, Szmida E, Karpiński P, Loska O, Sąsiadek MM, Frydecka D. Lower LINE-1 methylation in first-episode schizophrenia patients with the history of childhood trauma. Epigenomics. 2015;**7**(8):1275-1285. DOI: 10.2217/epi.15.68

[51] Schür RR, van Leeuwen JMC, Houtepen LC, et al. Glucocorticoid receptor exon 1_Fmethylation and the cortisol stress response in health and disease. Psychoneuroendocrinology. 2018;**97**:182-189. DOI: 10.1016/j.psyneuen.2018.07.018

[52] Meghani SH, Buck HG, Dickson VV, et al. The conceptualization and measurement of comorbidity: A review of the interprofessional discourse. Nursing Research & Practice. 2013;**2013**:192782. DOI: 10.1155/2013/192782

[53] van Weel C, Schellevis FG. Comorbidity and guidelines: Conflicting interests. Lancet. 2006;**367**(9510):550-551. DOI: 10.1016/S0140-6736(06)68198-1

[54] Insel TR. Rethinking schizophrenia. Nature. 2010;**468**(7321):187-193. DOI: 10.1038/nature09552

[55] Insel TR, Cuthbert B, Garvey M, Heinssen R, Pine DS, Quinn K, et al. Research domain criteria (RDoC): Toward a new classification framework for research on mental disorders. American Psychiatric Association. 2010;**167**(7):748-751. DOI: 10.1176/appi.ajp.2010.09091379

[56] Panov G. Dissociative model in patients with resistant schizophrenia. Frontiers in Psychiatry. 2022;**13**:845493. DOI: 10.3389/fpsyt.2022.845493

[57] Nakata Y, Kanahara N, Kimura A, et al. Autistic traits and cognitive profiles of treatment-resistant schizophrenia. Schizophrenia Research Cognition. 2020;**22**:100186. DOI: 10.1016/j.scog.2020.100186

[58] Lord C, Rutter M, Le Couteur A. Autism Diagnostic Interview-Revised: A revised version of a diagnostic interview for caregivers of individuals with possible pervasive developmental disorders. Journal of Autism and Developmental Disorders. 1994;**24**(5):659-685. DOI: 10.1007/BF02172145

[59] Lord C, Rutter M, DiLavore PC, Risi S, Gotham K, Bishop S. Autism Diagnostic Observation Schedule. Torrance, CA: Western Psychological Services; 2012

[60] Weathers FW, Bovin MJ, Lee DJ, et al. The Clinician-Administered PTSD Scale for DSM-5 (CAPS-5): Development and initial psychometric evaluation in military veterans. Psychological Assessment. 2018;**30**(3):383-395. DOI: 10.1037/pas0000486

[61] Lovaas OI. Behavioral treatment and normal educational and intellectual functioning in young autistic children. Journal of Consulting and Clinical Psychology. 1987;**55**(1):3-9. DOI: 10.1037//0022-006x.55.1.3

[62] Mesibov GB. Program for child with autism. Journal of Autism and Developmental Disorders. 2004;**34**(3):363. DOI: 10.1023/b:jadd.0000029673.75348.6a

[63] Oral R, Ramirez M, Coohey C, et al. Adverse childhood experiences and trauma informed care: The future of health care. Pediatric Research. 2016;**79**(1-2):227-233. DOI: 10.1038/pr.2015.197

[64] Hayes AM, Yasinski C, Grasso D, et al. Constructive and unproductive processing of traumatic experiences in trauma-focused cognitive-behavioral therapy for youth. Behavior Therapy. 2017;**48**(2):166-181. DOI: 10.1016/j.beth.2016.06.004

[65] Cohen JA, Mannarino AP. Trauma-focused cognitive behavioral therapy for childhood traumatic separation. Child Abuse & Neglect. 2019;**92**:179-195. DOI: 10.1016/j.chiabu.2019.03.006

Chapter 7

Clinical and Psychopathological Phenomenology of Mild Acute Drug-Induced Akathisia

Victor Obyedkov, Oleg Gorgun, Alexandr Hodjaev, Tatsiana Dakukina, Irina Hvostova, Yulia Kaminskaya, Siarhei Osipchyk, Fedor Khlebokazov, Vera Ivanitskaya, Olga Lapysh and Aliaksandra Kuchynskaya

Abstract

The study is devoted to the clinical and psychopathological phenomenology of mild acute drug-induced akathisia that occurs in the treatment of schizophrenia. The relationship between clinical symptoms and features of neurocognitive status with acute drug-induced akathisia resulting from the appointment of standardized antipsychotic therapy to patients was studied. It was found that patients with paranoid schizophrenia with mild acute drug-induced akathisia have more pronounced general psychopathological symptoms, such as anxiety, tension, depression, refusal to cooperate, weakening of impulsivity control, and congestion of mental experiences. According to the assessment of the risk profile of aggression, additional symptoms are more pronounced, such as anger, difficulties in delaying gratification (delayed reward), and affective lability. According to the results of the study of the neurocognitive status, markers of mild acute drug-induced akathisia were identified: impaired stability of active attention, impaired working memory, decreased automation of thinking, and impaired executive functions.

Keywords: schizophrenia, acute drug-induced akathisia, psychopathological symptoms, neurocognitive status

1. Introduction

Schizophrenia is a disease that exerts a significant economic cost in terms of loss of the patient's ability to work, destruction of social ties, and critically reducing the quality of life [1]. Medical care for paranoid schizophrenia is not devoid of controversial and problematic issues that require careful consideration and comprehensive analysis [2]. One of them is the issue of timely diagnosis of acute drug-induced akathisia. The American Psychiatric Association's Diagnostic and statistical manual of mental disorders (DSM-5) describes medication-induced acute akathisia as subjective complaints of restlessness, often accompanied by observed excessive movements (e.g., fidgety movements of the legs, rocking from foot to foot, pacing, and inability to sit or stand still), developing within a few weeks of starting or raising the dosage of a medication (such as neuroleptic), or after reducing the dosage of a medication used to treat extrapyramidal symptoms. Rocking, pacing, shifting weight while standing, and an inability to remain seated are commonly observed clinically [3].

There are no clear recent data on the prevalence of akathisia. Akathisia may appear as a side effect of prolonged use of antipsychotic drugs. From 15–45% of people taking antipsychotic drugs experience akathisia [4, 5].

Since it is known that this occurs as a result of the treatment of a mental disorder, the timely recognition of akathisia is of key importance [6]. Correction and treatment of drug-induced extrapyramidal disorders (EPR), which include akathisia, begin with a statement of their pronounced nature, the main sign of which is their obvious motor component. However, after reaching the degree of severity, acute drug-induced akathisia tends to become chronic, despite the recommended methods of correction [7]. Pronounced acute drug-induced akathisia often leads the patient to the decision to abandon the recommended treatment regimens [8], aggravates the psychotic and affective symptoms of the underlying disease [9, 10], and almost always worsens the quality of life of patients [11, 12]. The appearance of signs of akathisia in the patient negatively affects labor and social activity [13] and leads to additional social stigmatization [11].

The main problem with timely detection of acute drug-induced akathisia is that before the stage of development of pronounced motor manifestations, it is manifested by psychopathological symptoms that have an external similarity with some symptoms of schizophrenia, often taken by doctors as symptoms of the disease and regarded as a worsening of the underlying disease [14]. Acute drug-induced akathisia is often manifested only by a subjective feeling of unexplained anxiety and internal anxiety, which can be regarded by a doctor as an exacerbation of the underlying disease and lead to an erroneous decision to increase the dose of the prescribed antipsychotic, which in turn enhances akathisia [8].

The relevance of the study lies in the absence of reliable clinical and psychopathological markers for the diagnosis of mild acute drug-induced akathisia, which manifests itself in the actual provision of assistance after the occurrence of its pronounced motor manifestations when their correction itself counter-productively leads to additional adverse reactions from corrective medications [15, 16].

The aim of this study is to identify the clinical features and neurocognitive profile of patients with paranoid schizophrenia and mild acute drug-induced akathisia.

2. Materials and methods

Study design: open, observational, and cross-sectional study with directed formation of comparison groups. The comparison groups were congruent by gender ($\chi2 = 0.899$; $p = 0.638$), age ($F = 2.773$; $p = 0.064$), family ($\chi2 = 4.782$; $p = 0.572$), social ($\chi2 = 13.789$; $p = 0.063$) status, and level of education ($\chi2 = 9.330$; $p = 0.501$).

The object of the study was 333 patients (171 men, 162 women; average age 36.8 ± 11.71) with paranoid schizophrenia (F20.09, F20.01, F20.00, F20.02, F20.03 according to ICD10) undergoing inpatient treatment at the state institution "Republican Research and Practice Center for Mental Health" (Minsk, Belarus). All patients at the time of the study were taking antipsychotic drug therapy in accordance with the protocol for the diagnosis and treatment of mental and behavioral disorders [17]. Informed consent to participate in the study was signed by all participants of the study.

Diagnosis of clinical symptoms of schizophrenia was carried out using the PANSS scale [18].

To assess the severity of early drug-induced extrapyramidal symptoms, the extrapyramidal symptoms rating scale (ESRSA) was used [19].

The main group included patients with schizophrenia who, at the time of the study, had only mild acute drug-induced akathisia (group A), which, according to the guidelines for the use of the ESRS-A scale [19], is characterized by subjective complaints of the patient about a feeling of anxiety or a desire to move, with which, it is possible to cope that do not affect the patient's daily activity and manifest themselves less than 50% of the time, as well as objective little-expressed restless movements when the patient feels the need to move at least one limb, which manifests themselves less than 50% of the patient's observation time. Scores on the subscales of the ESRS scale N (parkinsonism) = 0, A (akathisia) = 1–2, D (dystonia) = 0, DK (dyskinesia) = 0. The comparison group consisted of patients with neuroleptic parkinsonism (NP) (group B), which is characterized by resistance to passive movements in the upper extremities, lower extremities or neck; low amplitude tremor of the face, jaws, lips, head, upper limbs or hands, lower limbs or feet during movement or postural tremor (observed periodically less than 50% of the time, absent at rest); slight decrease in facial expression, hypomimia; slight decrease in friendly hand movements, slight stoop posture; latero-, antero- or retropulsion in which the patient regains balance without assistance; moderately slow movements, weak impoverishment of movements. Estimates by subscales of the ESRS scale N = 1–2, A = 0, D = 0, and DC = 0. The control group consisted of patients with paranoid schizophrenia without extrapyramidal disorders: scores on the subscales of the ESRS scale N = 0, A = 0, D = 0, and DC = 0.

Inclusion criteria: The main group (n = 127) included patients with schizophrenia who had acute drug-induced akathisia at the time of the study; (group A): scores on the ESRS scale subscales N (parkinsonism) = 0, A (akathisia) = 1–2, D (dystonia) = 0, DK (dyskinesia) = 0, and total ESRS score = 1–2. The comparison group (n = 115) consisted of patients with neuroleptic parkinsonism (group B): scores on the subscales of the ESRS scale N = 1–2, A = 0, D = 0, DC = 0, and total ESRS score = 1–2. The control group (n = 91) consisted of patients with paranoid schizophrenia without extrapyramidal disorders: scores on the subscales of the ESRS scale N = 0, A = 0, D = 0, DK = 0, and total ESRS score = 0.

The criteria for excluding patients from the sample were: the presence of acute psychotic symptoms in the patient (on the PANSS scale and the sum of positive symptoms >30 points), pronounced manifestations of a personality defect (on the PANSS scale and the sum of negative symptoms >35 points), scores on the subscales of the ESRS scale N > 2, A > 2,D > 0, DK > 0, total ESRS score > 2.

The comparison groups were congruent by gender ($\chi2$ = 0.899; p = 0.638), age (F = 2.773; p = 0.064), family ($\chi2$ = 4.782; p = 0.572), social ($\chi2$ = 13.789; p = 0.063) status, level of education ($\chi2$ = 9.330; p = 0.501).

The cognitive sphere of the patients under study was assessed using the following techniques: Schulte tables; Luria test for auditory memorization of 10 and unrelated words; visual memorization test for 10 and unrelated words; trail-making test (TMT); Stroop color-word interference test; and Wisconsin card sorting test (WCST).

The data were processed on a personal computer using the SPSS 20.0 statistical package.

3. Results and discussion

When conducting a one-factor analysis of variance, it was found that there were no differences in any of the clusters of positive symptoms in the comparison groups (ANOVA, $p > 0.05$).

It was found that there were significant differences in the severity of negative symptoms in the comparison groups (total score of negative symptoms, ANOVA, $F = 26.09$; $p = 0.001$). These differences occurred due to clusters H1 blunted affect (ANOVA, $F = 29.14$; $p = 0.001$) and H2 emotional detachment (ANOVA, $F = 22.09$; $p = 0.006$). For other negative symptoms, no differences were found in the groups during comparison (ANOVA, $F < 3.0$; $p > 0$). (**Table 1**).

In a pairwise comparison, it was found that the negative symptoms in group A patients did not differ from those in the control group (post hoc analysis, LSD, and $p > 0.05$). Blunted affect and emotional detachment were statistically more pronounced in group B patients compared to group A and control group patients (post hoc analysis, LSD, and $p < 0.05$) (**Table 2**).

It was found that there were significant differences in the severity of general psychopathological symptoms in the comparison groups (total score of general psychopathological symptoms, ANOVA, $F = 25.92$; $p = 0.001$).

These differences occurred due to clusters O2 anxiety (ANOVA, $F = 31.09$; $p < 0.001$) and O4 tension (ANOVA, $F = 12.82$; $p = 0.04$), O6 - depression (ANOVA, $F = 28.78$; $p < 0.001$), O8 - refusal to cooperate (ANOVA, $F = 9.34$; $p = 0.001$), O14 - weakening of impulsivity control (ANOVA, $F = 27.23$; $p = 0.001$), O15 - congestion of mental experiences (ANOVA, $F = 19.26$; $p = 0.004$). For other common psychopathological symptoms, no differences were found in the comparison groups (ANOVA, $F = 2.8$; $p > 0.05$) (**Table 3**).

In a pairwise comparison, it was found that the group of patients with acute drug-induced akathisia (group A) differs from patients with neuroleptic parkinsonism (group B) and groups without extrapyramidal disorders (control group) with statistically more pronounced following signs: anxiety (O2), tension (O3), depression (O4), refusal to cooperation (O8), weakening of impulsivity control (O14), and workload with mental experiences (O15) (post hoc analysis, LSD, and $p < 0.05$). For other common psychopathological symptoms, no differences were found in the comparison groups (post hoc analysis, LSD, and $p > 0.05$) (**Table 4**).

It was found that there were significant differences in the severity of additional symptoms in the three compared groups ($F = 29.25$; $p = 0.001$).

Negative symptoms on the PANSS scale	Statistical significance of differences	
H1 - blunted effect	F = 29,14	p = 0,001
H2 - emotional detachment	F = 22,09	p = 0,006
H3 - difficulties in communication	F = 2,19	p = 0,09
H4 - passive-apathetic social withdrawal	F = 2,85	p = 0,07
H5 – violation of abstract thinking	F = 1,94	p = 0,12
H6 – violation of spontaneity and smooth thinking	F = 2,90	p = 0,06
H7 - stereotypical thinking	F = 2,1	p = 0,1

Table 1.
Intergroup differences in negative symptoms (ANOVA and p-significance level).

Comparison groups	***H1 - blunted affect***			***H2 - emotional detachment***			***H3 - communication difficulties***		
	Group A, M = 1,75	**Group B, M = 5,01**	**Control group, M = 1,20**	**Group A, M = 2,09**	**Group B, M = 5,08**	**Control group, M = 2,20**	**Group A, M = 3,71**	**Group B, M = 3,12**	**Control group, M = 3,75**
Group A		0,01	0,12		0,04	0,41		0,14	0,14
Group B	0,01		0,04	0,04		<0,001	0,14		0,75
Control group	0,12	0,04		0,41	<0,001		0,14	0,75	

Comparison groups	*H4 - passive-apathetic social isolation*			*H5 - violation of abstract thinking*			*H6 - violation of spontaneity and smooth thinking*			*H7 – stereotypical thinking*		
	Group A, M = 3,75	Group B, M = 4,01	Control group, M = 3,20	Group A, M = 3,09	Group B, M = 3,08	Control group, M = 3,36	Group A, M = 2,71	Group B, M = 2,12	Control group, M = 2,75	Group A, M = 2,71	Group B, M = 3,12	Control group, M = 2,75
Group A		0,49	0,10		0,25	0,16		0,24	0,24		0,16	0,16
Group B	0,49		0,34	0,25		0,17	0,24		0,75	0,16		0,75
Control group	0,10	0,34		0,16	0,17		0,24	0,75		0,16	0,75	

Table 2.
Intergroup differences in negative symptoms (post hoc analysis, LSD, and p-significance level).

General psychopathological symptoms on the PANSS scale	Statistical significance of differences	
01 - somatic concern	**F = 2,17**	**p = 0,09**
02 - anxiety	F = 31,09	P < 0,001
03 - feeling guilty	F = 2,01	p = 0,11
04 - tension	F = 12,82	p = 0,04
05 - mannerism and posture	F = 1,94	p = 0,12
06 - depression	F = 28,78	p < 0,001
07 - motor retardation	F = 2,11	p = 0,1
08 - refusal to cooperate	F = 9,34	p = 0,01
09 - unusual content of thoughts	F = 2,23	p = 0,1
010 - disorientation	F = 1,79	p = 0,15
011 - attention disorder	F = 2,85	p = 0,07
012 - reduced criticality and awareness of the disease	F = 1,98	p = 0,12
013 - violations of the will	F = 1,75	p = 0,17
014 - weakening of impulsivity control	F = 27,23	p = 0,001
015 - preoccupation with mental experiences	F = 19,26	p = 0,004
016 - active social exclusion	F = 2,55	p = 0,07

Table 3.
Intergroup differences in general psychopathological symptoms (ANOVA and p-significance level).

These differences occurred due to all three clusters of additional symptoms: D1 anger (ANOVA, F = 27.34; p < 0.001), aD2 difficulty in delaying gratification (delayed gratification) (ANOVA, F = 22.15; p = 0.001), and D3 affective lability (ANOVA, F = 29.19; p < 0.001) (**Table 5**).

In a pairwise comparison, it was found that the group of patients with acute drug-induced akathisia (group A) differs from patients with neuroleptic parkinsonism (group B) and the group without extrapyramidal disorders (control group) by the following more pronounced signs: "anger" (D1), "difficulty in delaying ratification (delayed reward)" (D2) and "affective lability" (D3) (post hoc analysis, LSD, and p < 0.05) (**Table 6**).

Analysis of the data obtained during clinical examination and subsequent statistical processing reliably demonstrates mild acute drug-induced akathisia in patients with paranoid schizophrenia has its own clinico-psychopathological phenomenology comparable to the disease itself.

In patients with paranoid schizophrenia and mild acute drug-induced akathisia, general psychopathological symptoms are most pronounced: anxiety, tension, depression, refusal to cooperate, weakening of impulsivity control, and congestion with mental experiences (post hoc analysis, LSD, p < 0.05).

In patients with paranoid schizophrenia with mild acute drug-induced akathisia, additional symptoms are more pronounced according to the assessment of the risk profile of aggression: anger, difficulties in delaying gratification (delayed gratification), and affective lability (post hoc analysis, LSD, p < 0.05).

The study of neurocognitive functions also revealed the characteristic features of drug-induced akathisia.

Comparison groups	***O1 - somatic concern***			***O2 - anxiety***			***O3 - feeling guilty***		
	Group A M = 3,79	**Group B M = 2,01**	**Control group M = 1,21**	**Group A M = 5,25**	**Group B M = 2,01**	**Control group M = 1,20**	**Group A M = 2,70**	**Group B M = 3,11**	**Control group M = 2,73**
Group A		0,48	0,11		<0,001	<0,001		0,17	0,16
Group B	0,48		0,52	<0,001		0,08	0,17		0,75
Control group	0,11	0,52		<0,001	0,08		0,16	0,75	
Группы сравнения	*O4 tension*			*O5 mannerism and posture*			*O6 depression*		
	Group A, M = 5,09	Group B, M = 2,38	Control group, M = 2,21	Group A, M = 2,72	Group B, M = 3,13	Control group, M = 2,11	Group A, M = 5,01	Group B, M = 2,68	Control group, M = 1,67
Group A		0,04	<0,001		0,16	0,11		0,001	<0,001
Group B	0,04		0,42	0,16		0,06	0,001		0,06
Control group	<0,001	0,42		0,11	0,06		<0,001	0,06	
Comparison groups	*O7 motor retardation*			*O8 refusal to cooperate*			*O9 unusual content of thoughts*		
	Group A M = 2,75	Group B M = 4,01	Control group M = 3,20	Group A M = 4,91	Group B M = 2,28	Control group M = 1,90	Group A M = 3,71	Group B M = 2,12	Control group M = 2,05
Group A		0,29	0,34		0,04	<0,001		0,15	0,11
Group B	0,29		0,09	0,04		0,43	0,15		0,79
Control group	0,34	0,09		<0,001	0,43		0,11	0,79	
Comparison groups	*O10 - disorientation*			*O11 attention disorders*			*O12 reduced criticality and awareness of the disease*		
	Group A M = 3,62	Group B M = 2,25	Control group M = 2,01	Group A M = 3,62	Group B M = 3,55	Control group M = 2,41	Group A M = 3,65	Group B M = 1,50	Control group M = 2,48
Group A		0,17	0,11		0,87	0,15		0,11	0,53
Group B	0,17		0,78	0,87		0,16	0,11		0,36
Control group	0,11	0,78		0,15	0,16		0,53	0,36	

Comparison groups	***O1 - somatic concern***			***O2 - anxiety***			***O3 - feeling guilty***		
	Group A M = 3,79	**Group B M = 2,01**	**Control group M = 1,21**	**Group A M = 5,25**	**Group B M = 2,01**	**Control group M = 1,20**	**Group A M = 2,70**	**Group B M = 3,11**	**Control group M = 2,73**

Comparison groups	*O13 violations of the will*			*O14 weakening of impulsivity control*		
	Group A M = 2,81	Group B M = 3,34	Control group M = 2,17	Group A M = 5,19	Group B M = 1,38	Control group M = 2,20
Group A		0,45	0,30		<0,001	0,007
Group B	0,45		0,21	<0,001		0,22
Control group	0,30	0,21		0,007	0,22	
Comparison groups	*O15 preoccupation with mental experiences*			*O16 active social exclusion*		
	Group A M = 5,10	Group B M = 2,28	Control group M = 2,01	Group A M = 3,10	Group B M = 2,91	Control group M = 2,13
Group A		<0,001	0,008		0,67	0,16
Group B	<0,001		0,72	0,67		0,25
Control group	0,008	0,72		0,16	0,25	

Table 4.
Intergroup differences in common psychopathological symptoms (post hoc analysis, LSD, and p-significance level).

Additional symptoms on a scale PANSS	**Statistical significance of differences**	
D1 - anger	F = 27,34	P < 0,001
D2 - difficulties in delaying gratification	F = 22,15	P = 0,001
D3 - affective lability	F = 29,19	P < 0,001

Table 5.
Intergroup differences of additional symptoms (ANOVA and p-significance level).

When passing the Luria test for visual memorization of 10 unrelated words, it was revealed that there were significant differences in the volume of short-term visual memory in comparison groups (ANOVA, $F = 11.27$; $p = 0.01$).

When performing the Luria test for auditory memorization of 10 unrelated words, differences in performance indicators of auditory short-term memory was not detected in the comparison groups (ANOVA, $F = 2.03$; $p = 0.13$).

When performing the "Schulte table" technique in comparison groups, significant differences were revealed in such characteristics of attention as work efficiency (ANOVA, $F = 21.72$; $p = 0.001$), workability (ANOVA, $F = 22.09$; $p = 0.001$), and mental stability (ANOVA, $F = 24.01$; $p < 0.001$) (**Table 1**).

In a pairwise comparison it was found that the group of patients with acute drug-induced akathisia (group A) differs from patients with neuroleptic parkinsonism (group B) and differs from the group without extrapyramidal disorders (control group) by a more pronounced violation of mental stability (NP) (post hoc analysis, LSD, $p < 0.05$). In turn, the group of patients with neuroleptic parkinsonism (group B) differs from the group with acute drug-induced akathisia (group A), and the group without extrapyramidal disorders (control group) by pronounced violations of visual short-term memory and attention characteristics, such as work efficiency (WE) and workability (WA) (post hoc analysis, LSD, and $p < 0.05$). There were no differences in the performance of auditory short-term memory in the comparison groups (post hoc analysis, LSD, and $p > 0.05$) (**Table 7**).

When performing the trail-making test (TMT), significant differences were revealed in the comparison groups both in terms of test execution time (ANOVA, $F = 18.38$; $p = 0.003$) and in the number of errors made (ANOVA, $F = 19.12$; $p = 0.002$) (**Table 7**).

In a pairwise comparison, it was found that the group of patients with acute drug-induced akathisia (group A) differs from patients with neuroleptic parkinsonism (group B) and the group without extrapyramidal disorders (control group) by a large number of errors made when performing the working memory test (RP(t) (post hoc analysis, LSD, $p < 0.05$). In turn, the group of patients with neuroleptic parkinsonism (group B) differs from the group of patients with acute drug-induced akathisia (group A) and the group without extrapyramidal disorders (control group) by a greater time spent on the working memory test (RP (e) (post hoc analysis, LSD, and $p < 0.05$) (**Table 8**).

When performing the Stroop test in the comparison groups, there are significant differences both in terms of the execution time of the 2nd part of the test (ANOVA, $F = 21.34$; $p = 0.001$) and in the number of errors made when performing the 2nd part of the test (ANOVA, $F = 22.32$; $p = 0.001$).

Comparison groups	*D1 - anger*			*D2 - difficulties in delaying gratification*			*D3 - affective lability*		
	Group A M = 5,10	**Group B** M = 1,78	**Control group** M = 2,03	**Group A** M = 5,01	**Group B** M = 1,86	**Control group** M = 1,98	**Group A** M = 5,89	**Group B** M = 1,61	**Control group** M = 2,15
Group A		<0,001	0,007		<0,001	0,006		<0,001	<0,001
Group B	<0,001		0,31	<0,001		0,52	<0,001		0,12
Control group	0,007	0,31		0,006	0,52		<0,001	0,12	

Table 6.
Intergroup differences of additional features for assessing the risk profile of aggression (post hoc analysis, LSD, and p-significance level).

Neurocognitive functions	Statistical significance of differences	
OE - operational efficiency	F = 21,72	p = 0,001
WA - Workability	F = 22,09	P = 0,001
MT - mental toughness	F = 24,01	p < 0,001
WSTM - verbal short-term memory	F = 2,03	p = 0,13
STVM - short-term visual memory	F = 11,27	p = 0,01
WM(e) - working memory (test execution time)	F = 18,38	P = 0,003
WM(e) - working memory (number of errors)	F = 19,12	p = 0,002
CF - Cognitive flexibility (number of errors in part 2 of the Stroop test)	F = 21,34	p = 0,001
AS - automation style (time to complete part 2 of the Stroop test)	F = 22,32	p = 0,001

Table 7.
Intergroup differences in the characteristics of attention, short-term and working memory, cognitive flexibility, and automation (ANOVA and p-significance level).

In a pairwise comparison, it was found that the group of patients with acute drug-induced akathisia (group A) differs from patients with neuroleptic parkinsonism (group B) and groups without extrapyramidal disorders (control group) in the automation style (AS), which is manifested by a large number of mistakes made when performing the 2nd part of the Stroop test (post hoc-analysis, LSD, $p < 0.05$). In turn, the group of patients with neuroleptic parkinsonism (group B) differs from the group of patients with acute drug-induced akathisia (group A) and the group without extrapyramidal disorders (control group) with impaired cognitive flexibility (CF), which is revealed by the greater time spent on the 2nd part of the Stroop test (post hoc analysis, LSD, and $p < 0.05$) (**Table 8**).

In the study of performance functions based on the Wisconsin card sorting test (WTSC) in comparison groups, differences were revealed in such indicators as the number of perseverative (ANOVA, $F = 19.71$; $p = 0.003$) and non-perseverative errors (ANOVA, $F = 21.92$; $p = 0.001$), the number of cards for passing the first category (ANOVA, $F = 22.01$;$p = 0.001$), and the number of district errors (ANOVA, $F = 24.81$; $p < 0.001$) (**Table 9**).

In a pairwise comparison it was found that the group of patients with acute drug-induced akathisia (group A) differs from patients with neuroleptic parkinsonism (group B) and the group without extrapyramidal disorders (control group) by a large number of non-superseverative (NS) and distributive errors (DE) when performing WTSC (post hoc analysis, LSD, $p < 0.05$). In turn, the group of patients with neuroleptic parkinsonism (group B) differs from the group of patients with acute drug-induced akathisia (group A) and the group without extrapyramidal disorders (control group) by a large number of cards for passing the first category of WTSC (FC) and a large number of perseverative errors when performing WTSC (PE) (post hoc analysis, LSD, and $p < 0.05$) (**Table 10**).

Summing up the results of this study, we can say that patients with schizophrenia who have developed mild acute drug-induced akathisia have statistically proven neurocognitive disorders that differ in their structure. Markers of mild acute drug-induced akathisia are impaired stability of active attention, impaired working memory, decreased automation of thinking, and impaired executive functions due to

Patient groups	*P performance (efficiency factor)*			*WP work-in-progress (work-in-progress coefficient)*			*MT mental toughness (resilience coefficient)*		
	Group A M = 52,26	**Group B M = 60,13**	**Control group M = 46,29**	**Group A M = 1,33**	**Group B M = 1,48**	**Control group M = 1,23**	**Group A M = 1,89**	**GroupB M = 1,39**	**Control group M = 1,27**
Group A		0,001	0,09		0,04	0,12		0,04	<0,001
Group B	0,001		<0,001	0,04		<0,001	0,04		0,06
Control group	0,09	<0,001		0,12	<0,001		<0,001	0,06	
Patient groups	*VShM verbal short-term memory (number of words) group*			*VSM visual short-term memory (number of words)*			*WM(s) working memory (time in seconds)*		
	Group A, M = 5,34	Group B, M = 5,72	Control group, M = 5,49	Group, AM = 5,97	Group B, M = 5,57	Control group, M = 6,38	Group A, M = 202,90	Group B, M = 234,73	Control group, M = 193,98
Group A		0,07	0,10		0,08	0,11		0,03	0,12
Group B	0,07		0,33	0,08		0,003	0,03		<0,001
Control group	0,10	0,33		0,11	0,003		0,12	<0,001	
Patient groups	*WM(e) working memory (number of errors)*			*CF cognitive flexibility (number of errors)*			*AS automation style (time in seconds)*		
	Group A M = 6,98	Group B M = 6,04	Control group M = 5,73	Group A M = 6,50	Group B M = 5,25	Control group M = 4,61	Group A M = 106,31	Group B M = 134,05	Control group M = 95,94
Group A		0,01	<0,001		0,01	<0,001		0,001	0,06
Group B	0,01		0,06	0,01		0,09	0,001		<0,001
Control group	<0,001	0,06		<0,001	0,09		0,06	<0,001	

Note: Group A is a group with mild acute drug-induced akathisia, group B is a group with mild early neuroleptic parkinsonism, and control group is a group without extrapyramidal disorders.

Table 8.
Intergroup differences in the characteristics of attention, short-term and working memory, cognitive flexibility, and automation (post hoc analysis, LSD, and p-significance level).

Test performance characteristics WTSC	Statistical significance of differences	
FC - number of cards to pass the 1st category	F = 19,71	p = 0,003
PE - perseverative errors	F = 21,92	P = 0,001
NE - non-perseverative errors	F = 22,01	p = 0,001
DE - distributive errors	F = 24,81	P < 0,001

Table 9.
Intergroup differences in performing functions (ANOVA and p-significance level).

Patient groups	***CN number of cards to pass the 1st category***			***PE perseverative errors (errors caused by fixation on a previous task)***		
	Group A M = 10,79	**Group B M = 12,62**	**Control group M = 9,91**	**Group A M = 21,92**	**Group B M = 26,65**	**Control group M = 20,26**
Group A		0,01	0,12		0,04	0,07
Group B	0,01		<0,001	0,04		<0,001
Control group	0,12	<0,001		0,07	<0,001	
Patient groups	*NE non-perseverative errors (other errors)*			*DE distributive errors (card sorting errors without rules)*		
	Group A M = 21,22	Group B M = 18,26	M = 16,50	Group A M = 16,25	Group B M = 13,24	Control group M = 13,20
Group A		0,01	<0,001		<0,001	<0,001
Group B	0,01		0,07	<0,001		0,41
Control group	<0,001	0,07		<0,001	0,41	

Note: Group A is a group with mild acute drug-induced akathisia, group B is a group with mild early neuroleptic parkinsonism, and control group is a group without extrapyramidal disorders.

Table 10.
Intergroup differences in performance functions in comparison groups (post hoc analysis, LSD, and p-significance level).

high distractibility (post hoc analysis, LSD, $p < 0.05$). Significant differences in neurocognitive profiles in patients with neuroleptic parkinsonism and acute drug-induced akathisia indicate a different pathoplastic basis for these disorders. This is important not only in the differential diagnosis of these types of extrapyramidal disorders among themselves but also in the specifics of their treatment. The participation of various neurocognitive blocks in the brain supports this phenomenon and is clinically significant for the development of further research in terms of treatment and rehabilitation of patients with acute drug-induced akathisia. Also, based on the data obtained, in the absence of expressed manifestations of acute drug-induced akathisia, the study of neurocognitive functions can be an important additional diagnostic tool for these disorders.

4. Conclusions

In patients with schizophrenia and mild acute drug-induced akathisia, the clinical picture is dominated by tension, depression, refusal to cooperate, weakening of impulsivity control, workload with mental experiences, anger, difficulties in delaying gratification, and affective lability (post hoc analysis, LSD, $p < 0.05$). The neurocognitive sphere suffers the stability of active attention, working memory, automation of thinking, and performing functions (post hoc analysis, LSD, $p < 0.05$). Timely diagnosis of acute drug-induced akathisia by clinical and neuropsychological signs will improve the quality and effectiveness of treatment.

Acknowledgements

The authors would like to thank the patients who agreed to the publication of this article, as well as the staff of the psychiatric department who supported the management of cases in the state institution «Republican Research and Practice Center for Mental Health», Minsk, Belarus. The study was funded by the Ministry of Health of Belarus.

Conflict of interest

The authors declare no conflict of interest.

Author details

Victor Obyedkov[1], Oleg Gorgun[1], Alexandr Hodjaev[2], Tatsiana Dakukina[2]*, Irina Hvostova[2], Yulia Kaminskaya[2], Siarhei Osipchyk[2], Fedor Khlebokazov[2], Vera Ivanitskaya[2], Olga Lapysh[2] and Aliaksandra Kuchynskaya[2]

1 Belarusian State Medical University, Minsk, Belarus

2 The State Institution "Republican Research and Practice Center for Mental Health", Minsk, Belarus

*Address all correspondence to: polak0208@mail.ru

References

[1] Fiona JC, Ferrari AJ, Santomauro DF, Diminic S, Stockings E, Scott JG, et al. Global epidemiology and burden of schizophrenia: Findings from the global burden of disease study 2016. Schizophrenia Bulletin. 2018;**44**(6): 1195-1203

[2] Pringsheim T, Gardner D, Addington D, Martino D, Morgante F, Ricciardi L, et al. The assessment and treatment of antipsychotic-induced akathisia. Canadian Journal of Psychiatry. 2018;**63**(11):719-729

[3] American Psychiatric Association. Diagnostic and Statistical Manual of Mental Disorders. 5th ed. Arlington: American Psychiatric Association; 2013

[4] Poyurovsky M. Acute antipsychotic-induced akatisia revisited. The British Journal of Psychiatry. 2010, 2010; **196**(2):89-91

[5] Berna F, Misdrahi D, Boyer L, et al. Akathisia: Prevalence and risk factors in a community-dwelling sample of patients with schizophrenia. Results from the FACE-SZ dataset. Schizophrenia Research. 2015;**169**(1–3):255-261

[6] Salem H, Nagpal C, Pigott T, Teixeira AL. Revisiting antipsychotic-induced akathisia: Current issues and prospective challenges. Current Neuropharmacology. 2017;**15**(5):789-798

[7] Misdrahi D, Tessier A, Daubigney A, Meissner W, Schürho F, et al. Extrapyramidal side effects of antipsychotics: Prevalence and risk factors. Results from the national FACE-cohort cover title extrapyramidal side effects and antipsychotics. The Journal of Clinical Psychiatry. 2019;**80**(1):e1-10. DOI: 10.4088/JCP.18m12246.hal-02473295

[8] Peitl MV, Prološčić J, Blažević-Zelić S, et al. Symptoms of agitated depression and/or akathisia. Psychiatria Danubina. 2011;**23**(1):108-110

[9] Reid AM, JP MN, Murphy TK. Side-effects of SSRIs disrupt multimodal treatment for pediatric OCD in a randomized-controlled trial. Journal of Psychiatric Research. 2015;**71**:140-147

[10] Duncan EJ, Adler LA, Stephanides M, et al. Akathisia and exacerbation of psychopathology: A preliminary report. Clinical Neuropharmacology. 2000;**23**:169-173

[11] Temmingh H, Stein DJ. Anxiety in patients with schizophrenia: Epidemiology and management. CNS Drugs. 2015;**29**(10):819-832

[12] Seemuller F, Lewitzka U, Bauer M, et al. The relationship of Akathisia with treatment emergent suicidality among patients with firstepisode schizophrenia treated with haloperidol or risperidone. Pharmacopsychiatry. 2012;**45**(7): 292-296

[13] Kim JH, Byun HJ. Non-motor cognitive-perceptual dysfunction associated with drug-induced parkinsonism. Human Psychopharmacology. 2009;**24**(2): 129-134

[14] Nair CJ, Josiassen RC, Abraham G, et al. Does akathisia influence psychopathology inpsychotic patients treated with clozapine? Biological Psychiatry. 1999;**45**(10):1376-1383

[15] Jetwa K. Pharmacological management of antipsychotic-induced akathisia% An update and treatment algorithm. BJPsych Advances. 2015; **21**(5):342-344

[16] Horiguchi J, Nichimatsu O, Inami Y. Succtsssful treatment with clonazepam for neuroleptic-induced akathisia. Acta Psychiatrica Scandinavia. 2013;**80**: 106-107

[17] Клинический Протокол оказания медицинской помощи пациентам с психическими и поведенческими расстройствами. Приказ Министерства Здравоохранения Республики Беларусь № 1387 от 31.10.2010, стр. 107–108

[18] Kay SR, Fiszbein A, Opler LA. The positive and negative syndrome scale (PANSS) for schizophrenia. Schizophrenia Bulletin. 1987;**13**(2): 261-276

[19] Chouinard G, Ross-Chouinard A, Annable L, et al. Extrapyramidal rating scale. The Canadian Journal of Neurological Sciences. 1980;7:233-239